ELEANOR AND GERALDINE

ISBN: 9798306051352
Kindle Direct Publishing
Portland, Oregon
Copyright © 2025 James T. Rosenbaum, MD

ELEANOR AND GERALDINE

Written by **Jim Rosenbaum, MD**
Illustrated by **Doug Katagiri**

DEDICATED TO OUR FAMILIES:

Sandra, Lisa, Jennifer, Meredith, and Alex

Val, Ani, Steve, Zach, Amanda,
Ellie, Cara, Alden, and Tate

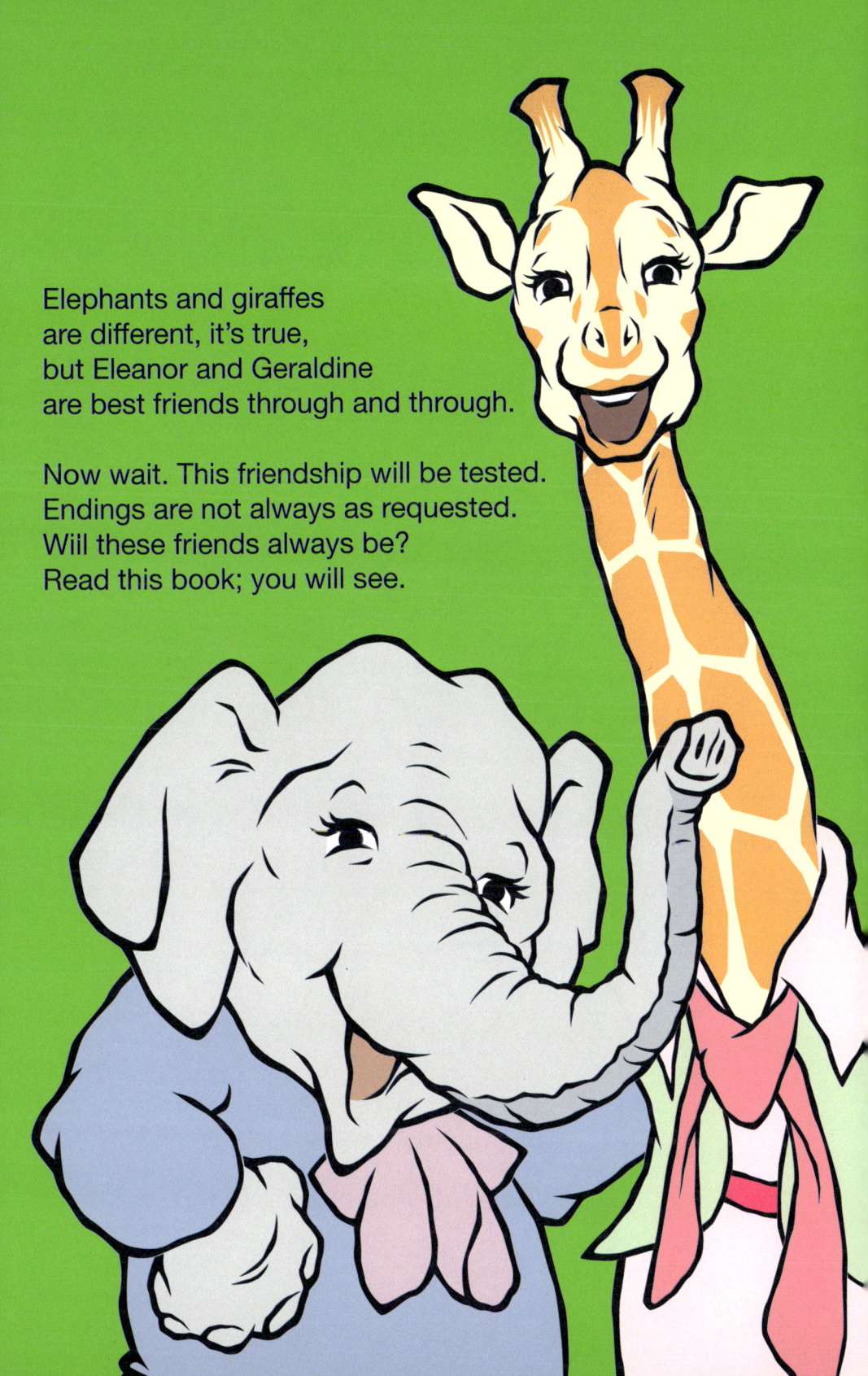

Elephants and giraffes
are different, it's true,
but Eleanor and Geraldine
are best friends through and through.

Now wait. This friendship will be tested.
Endings are not always as requested.
Wiil these friends always be?
Read this book; you will see.

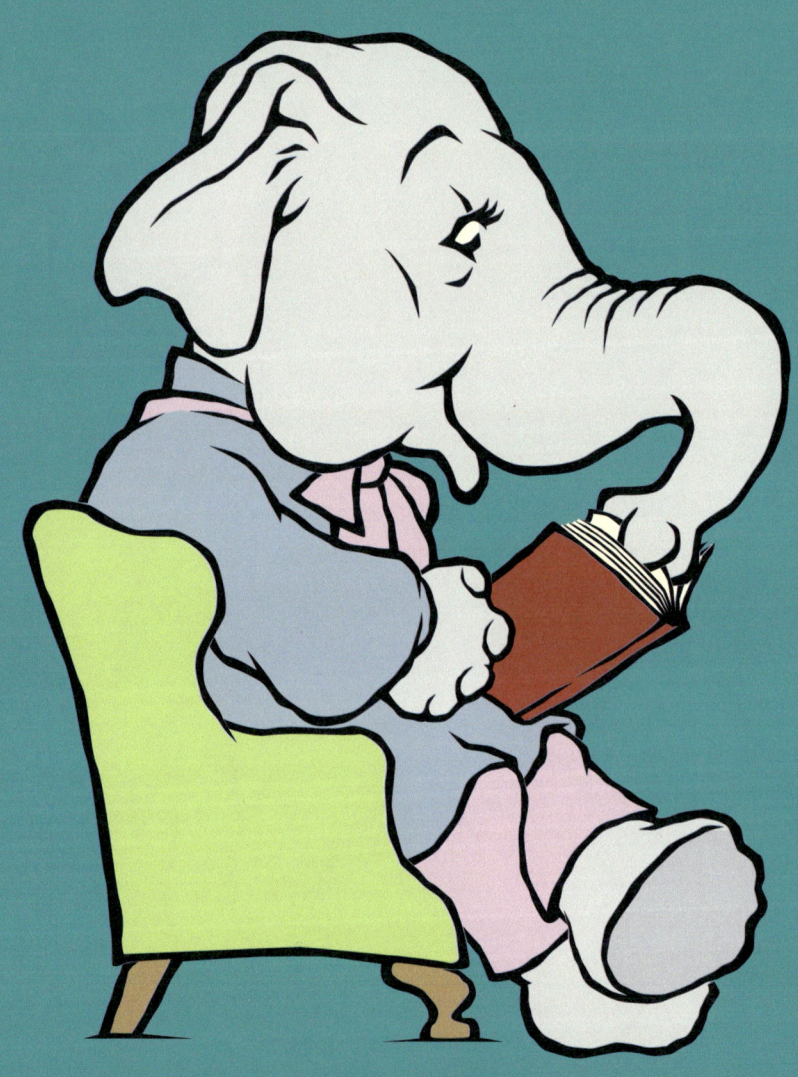

Ellie Elephant
Is reserved and serene,

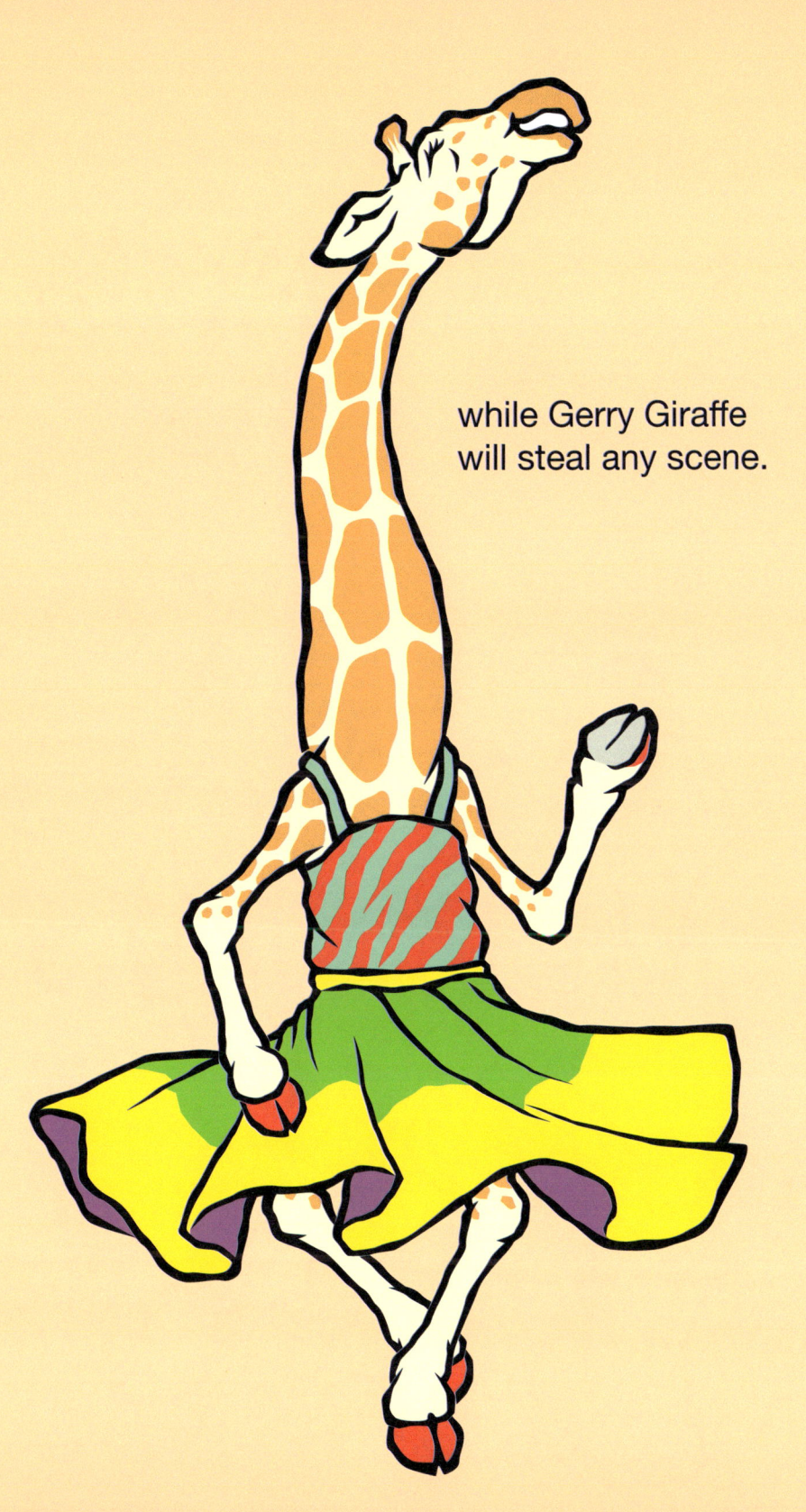

while Gerry Giraffe will steal any scene.

Together they stroll
along paths through the zoo

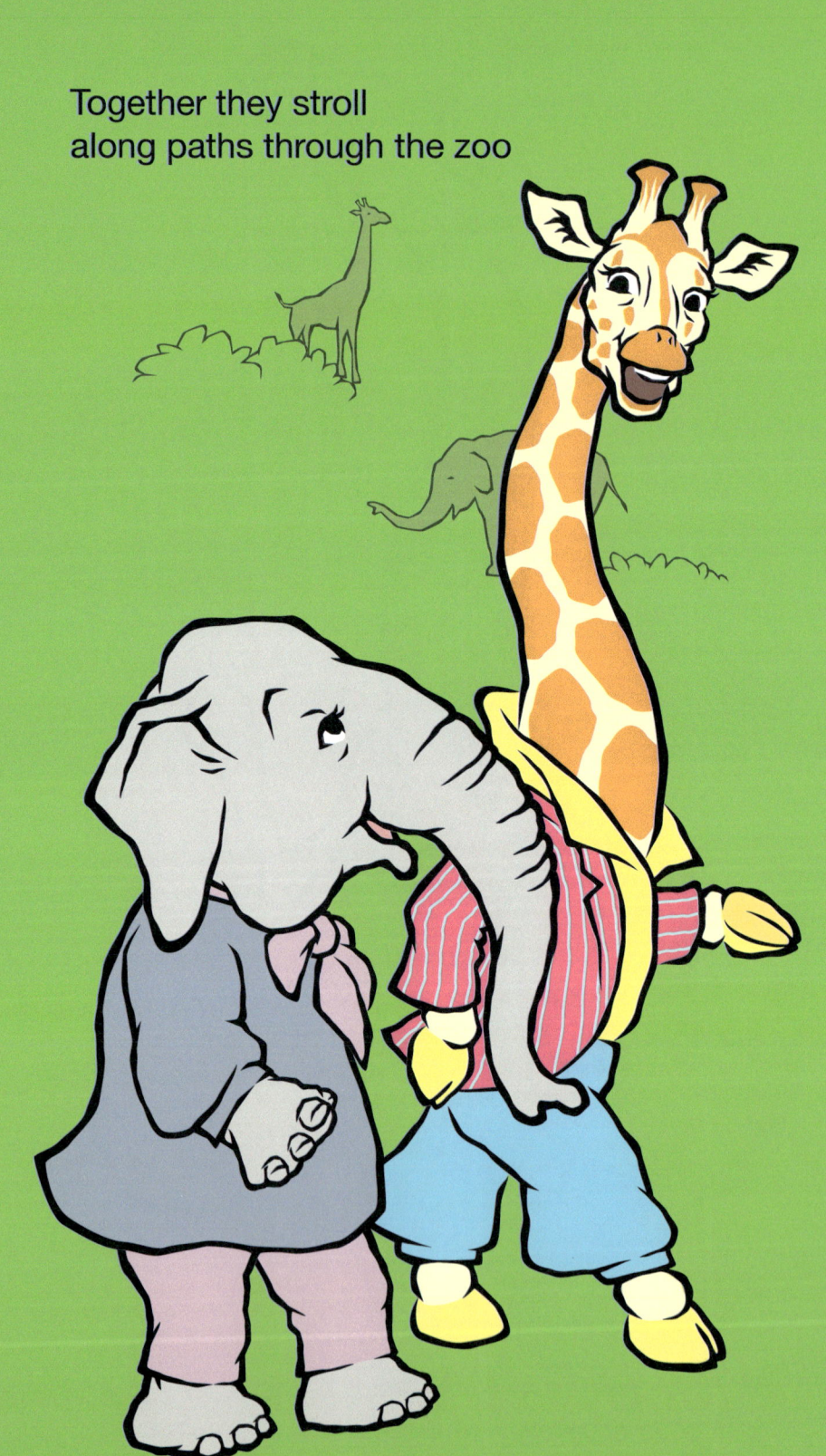

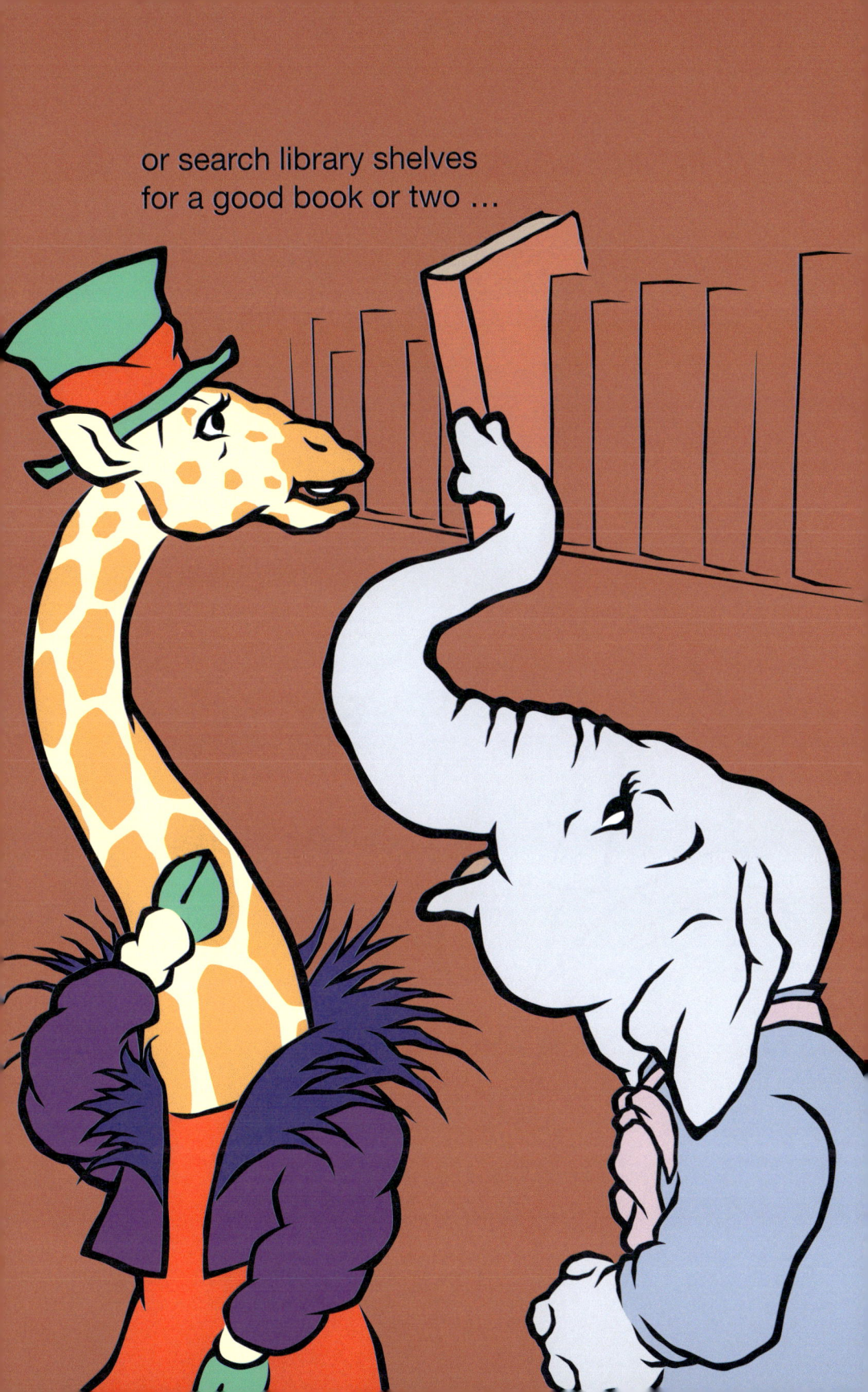

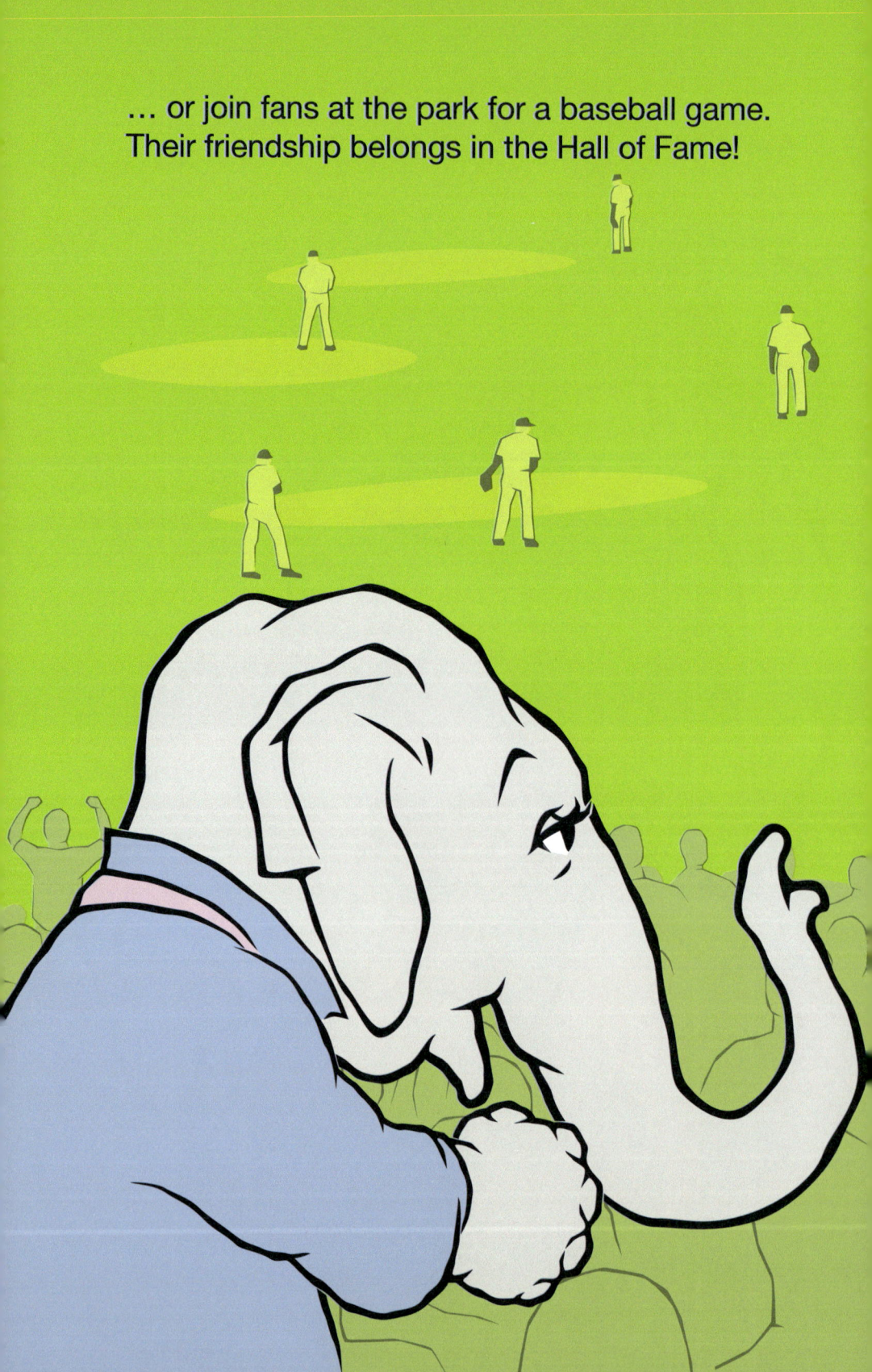

… or join fans at the park for a baseball game. Their friendship belongs in the Hall of Fame!

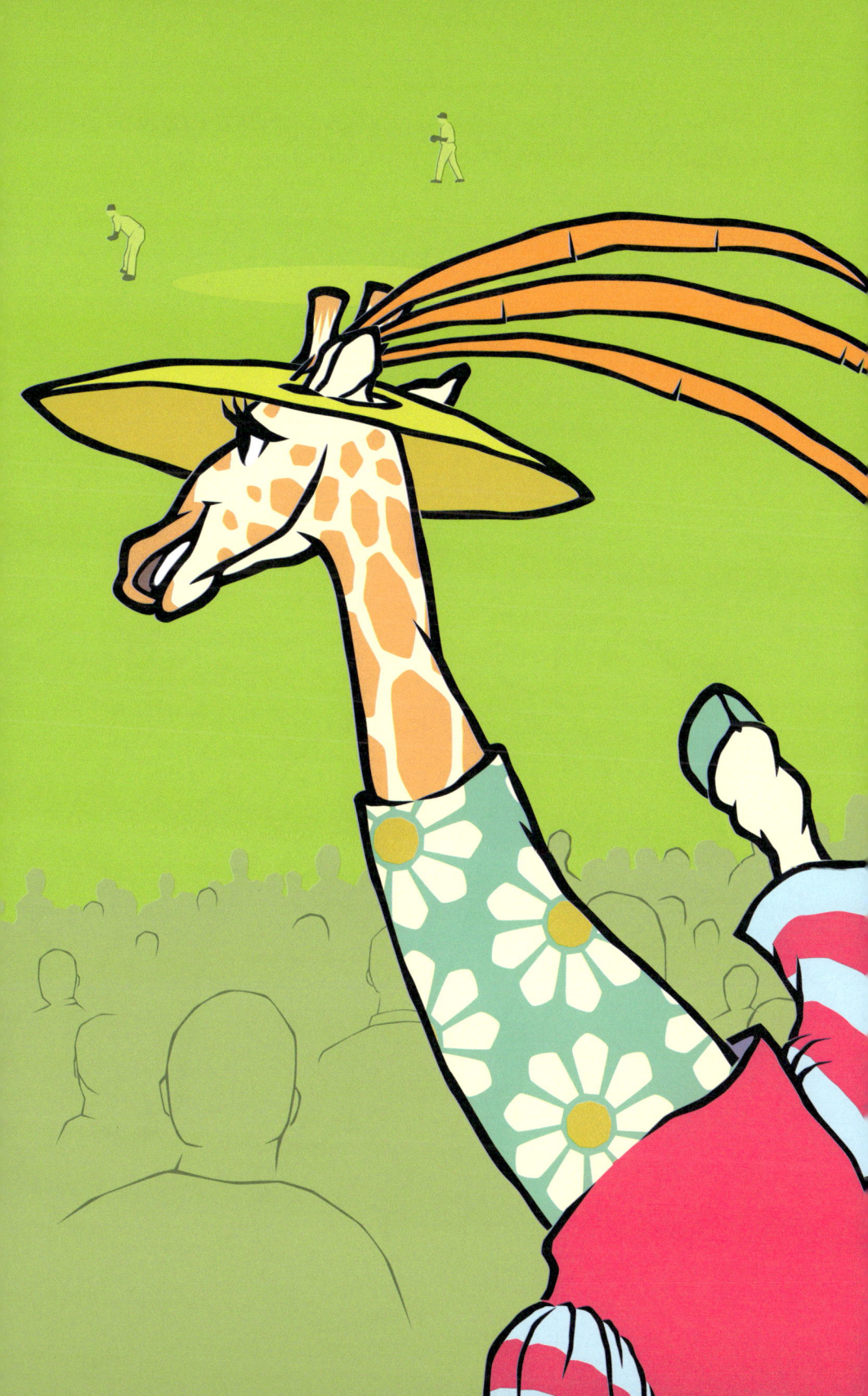

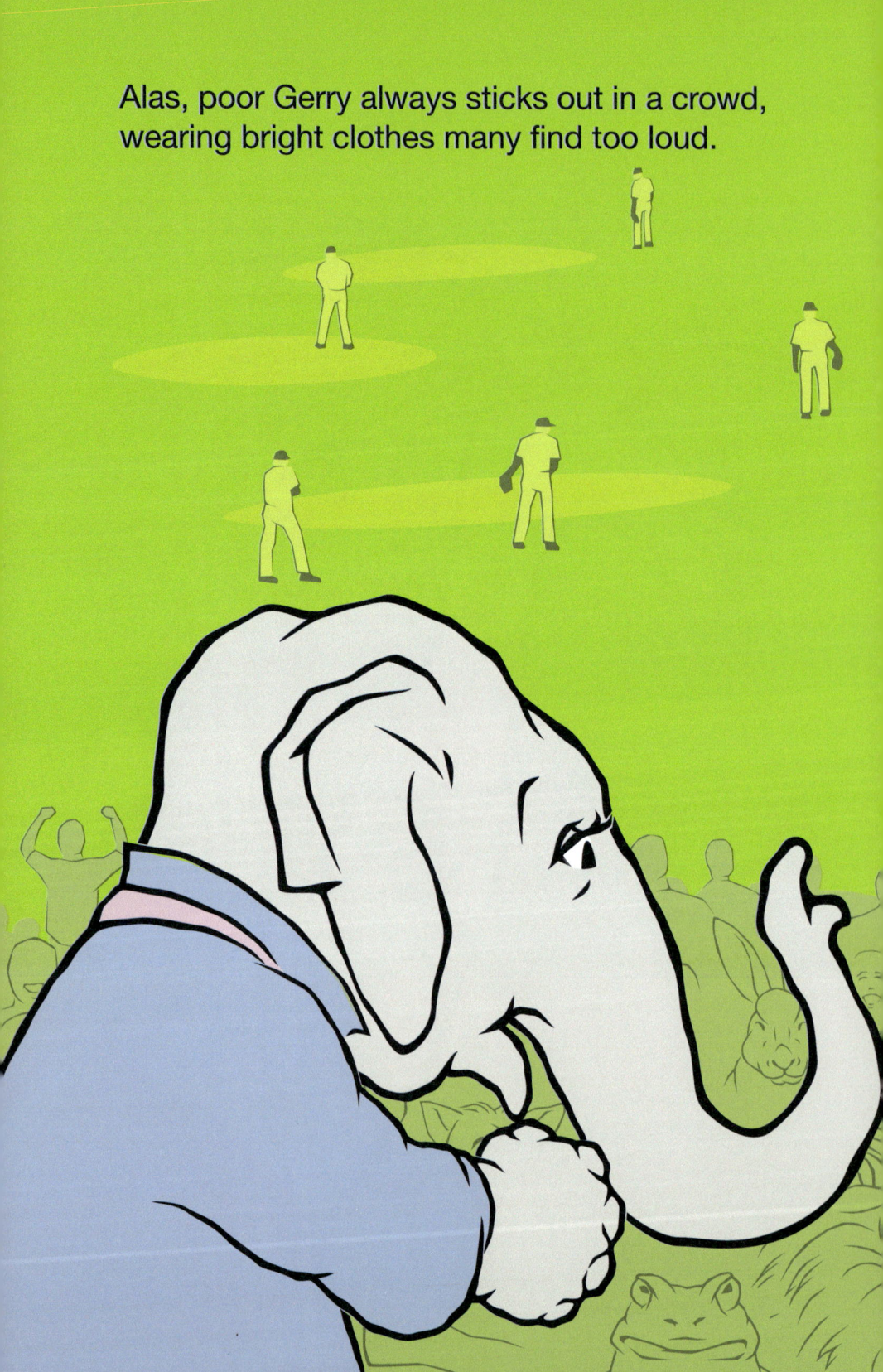

Alas, poor Gerry always sticks out in a crowd, wearing bright clothes many find too loud.

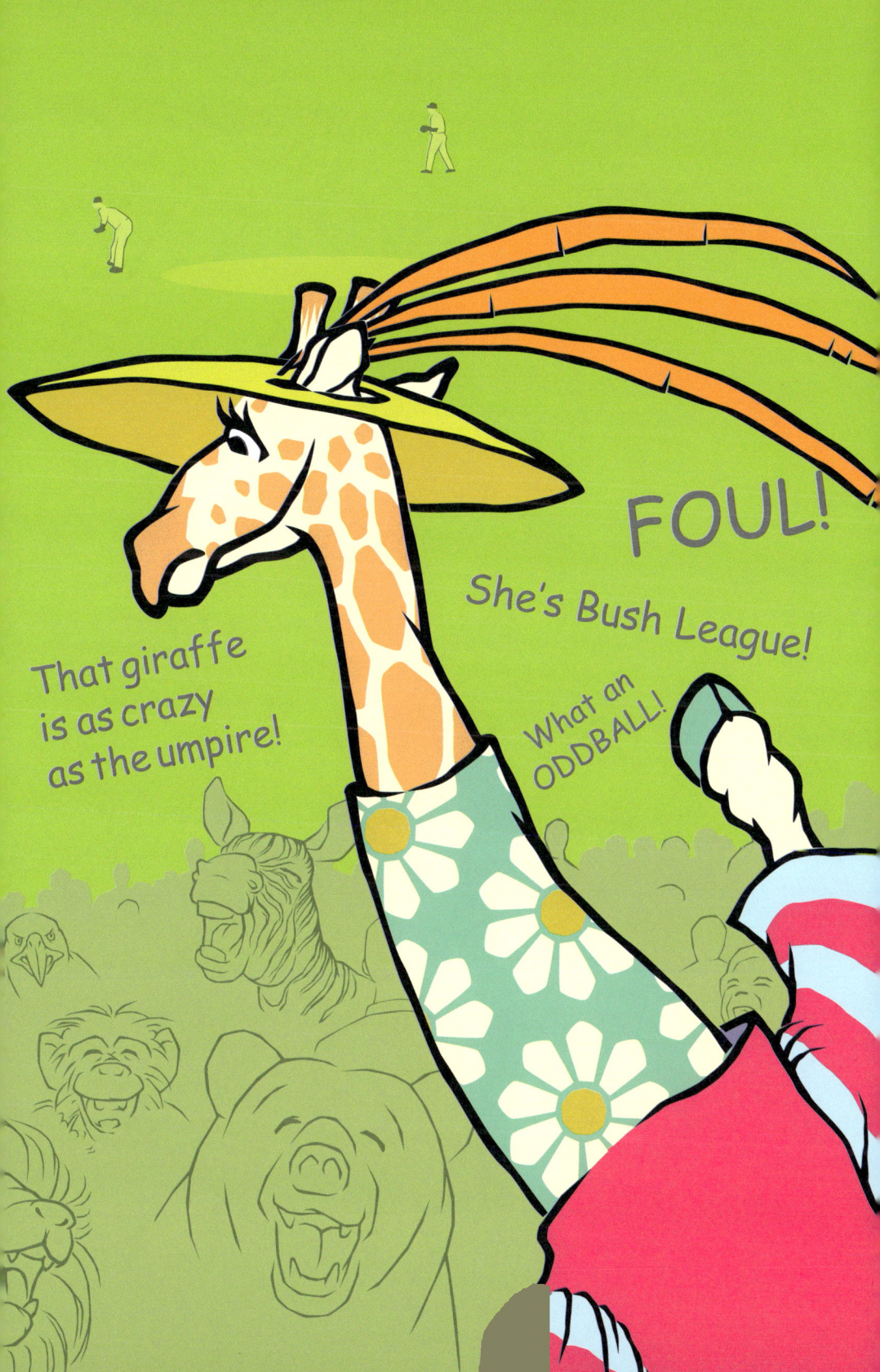

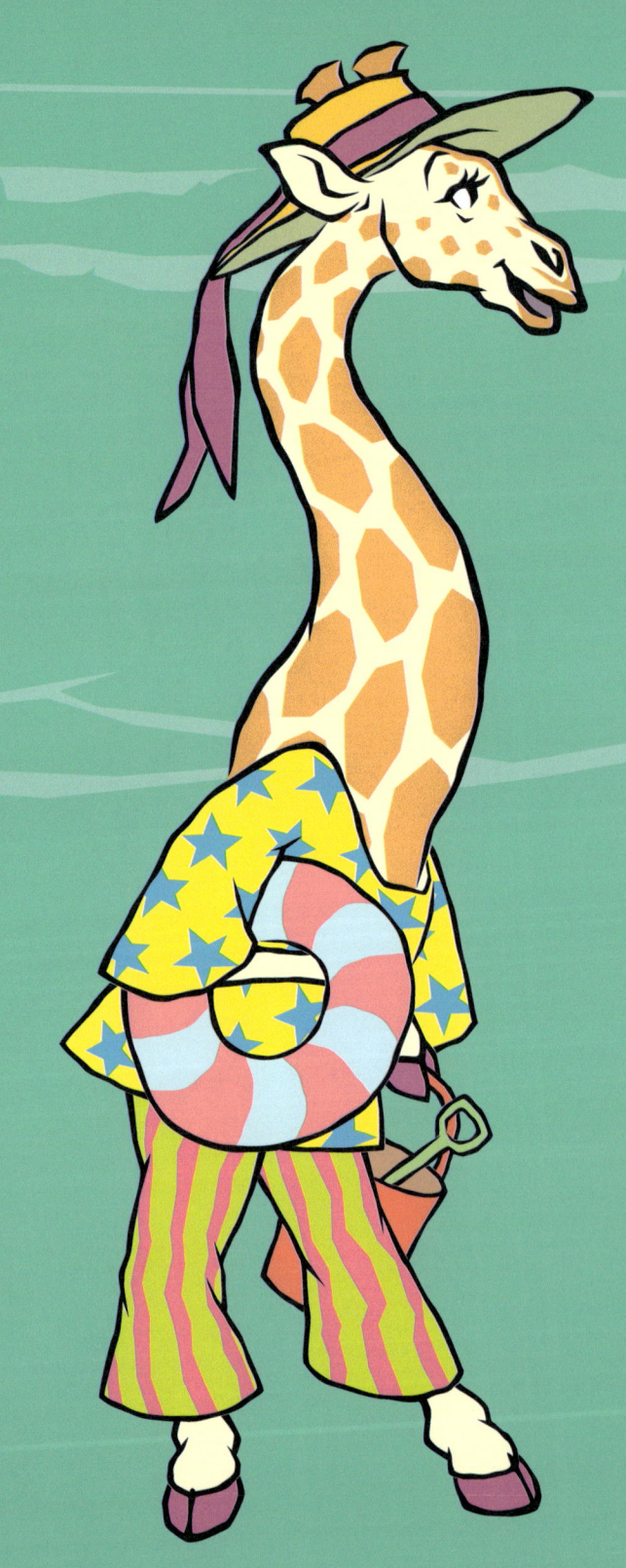

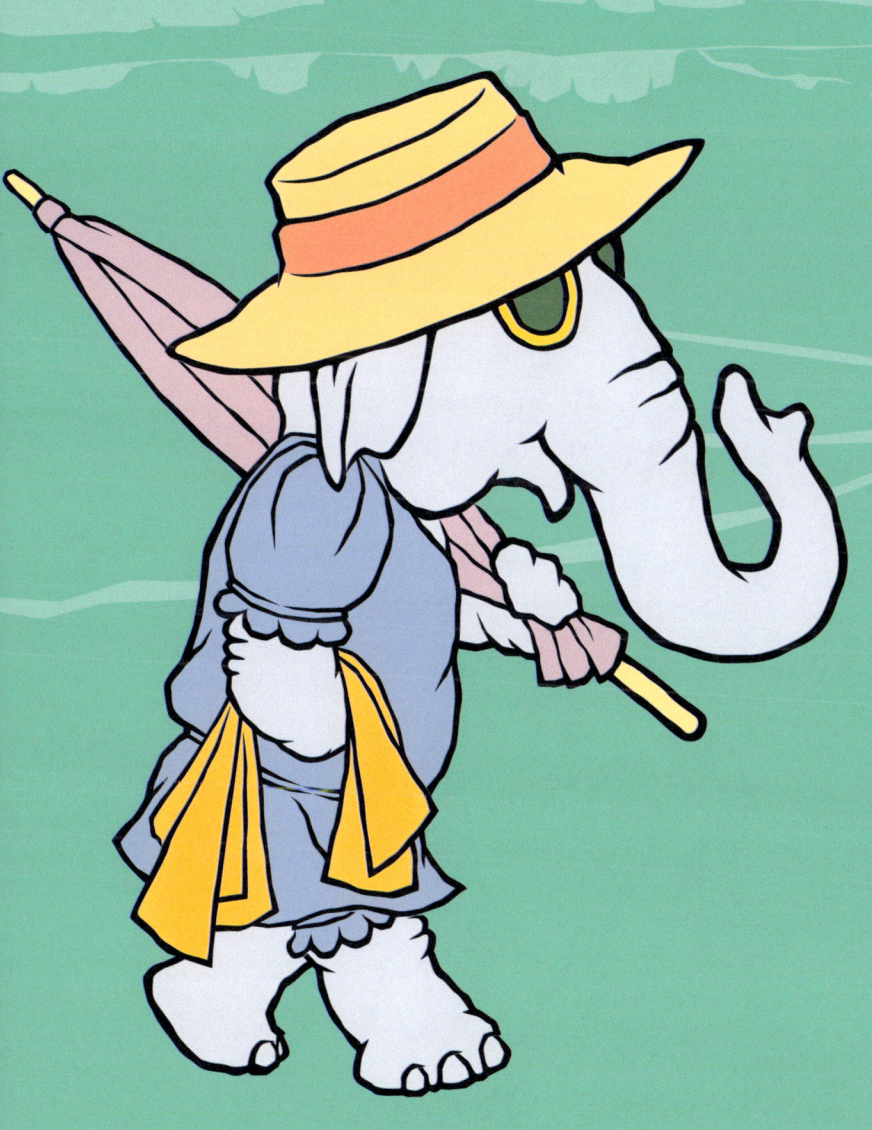

Off they go to the beach
for some surf and sand.

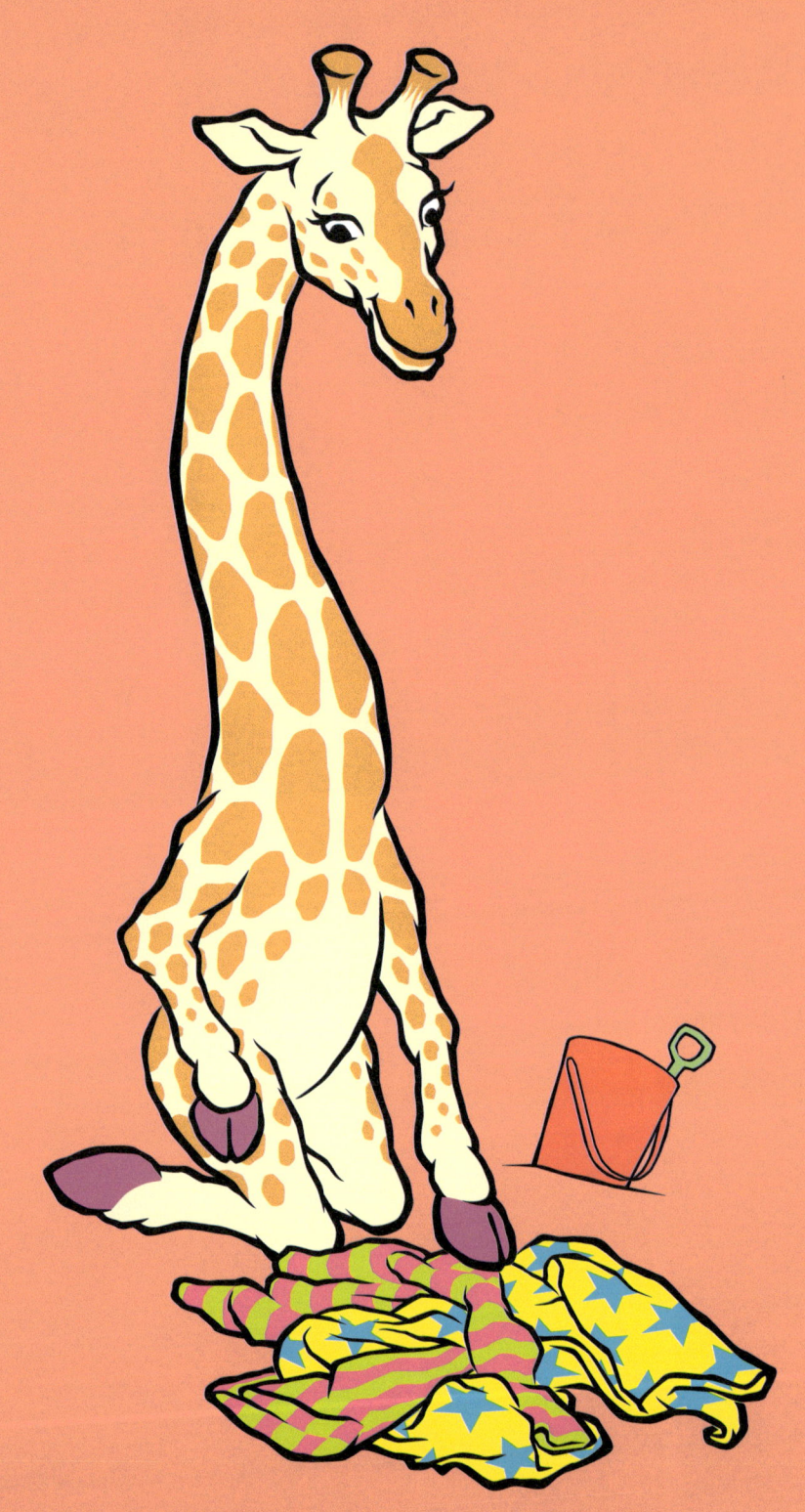

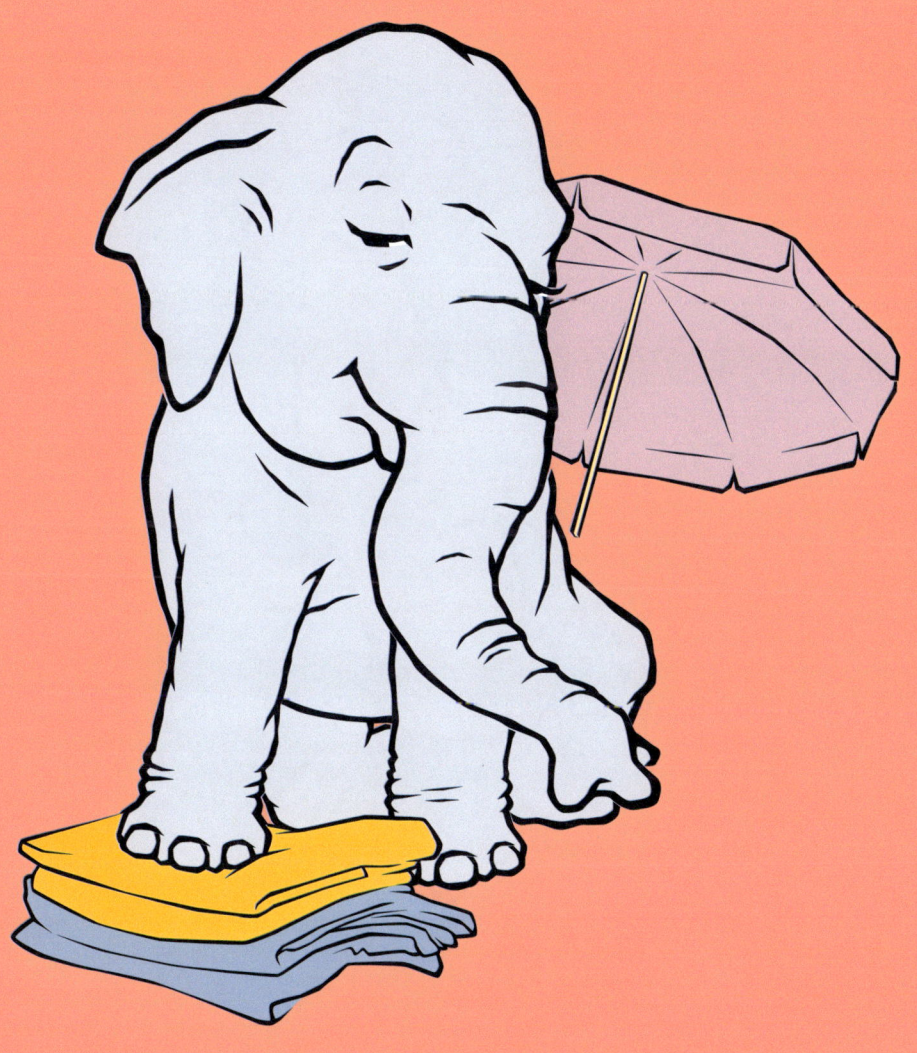

Off come their clothes
to stay safe on dry land.

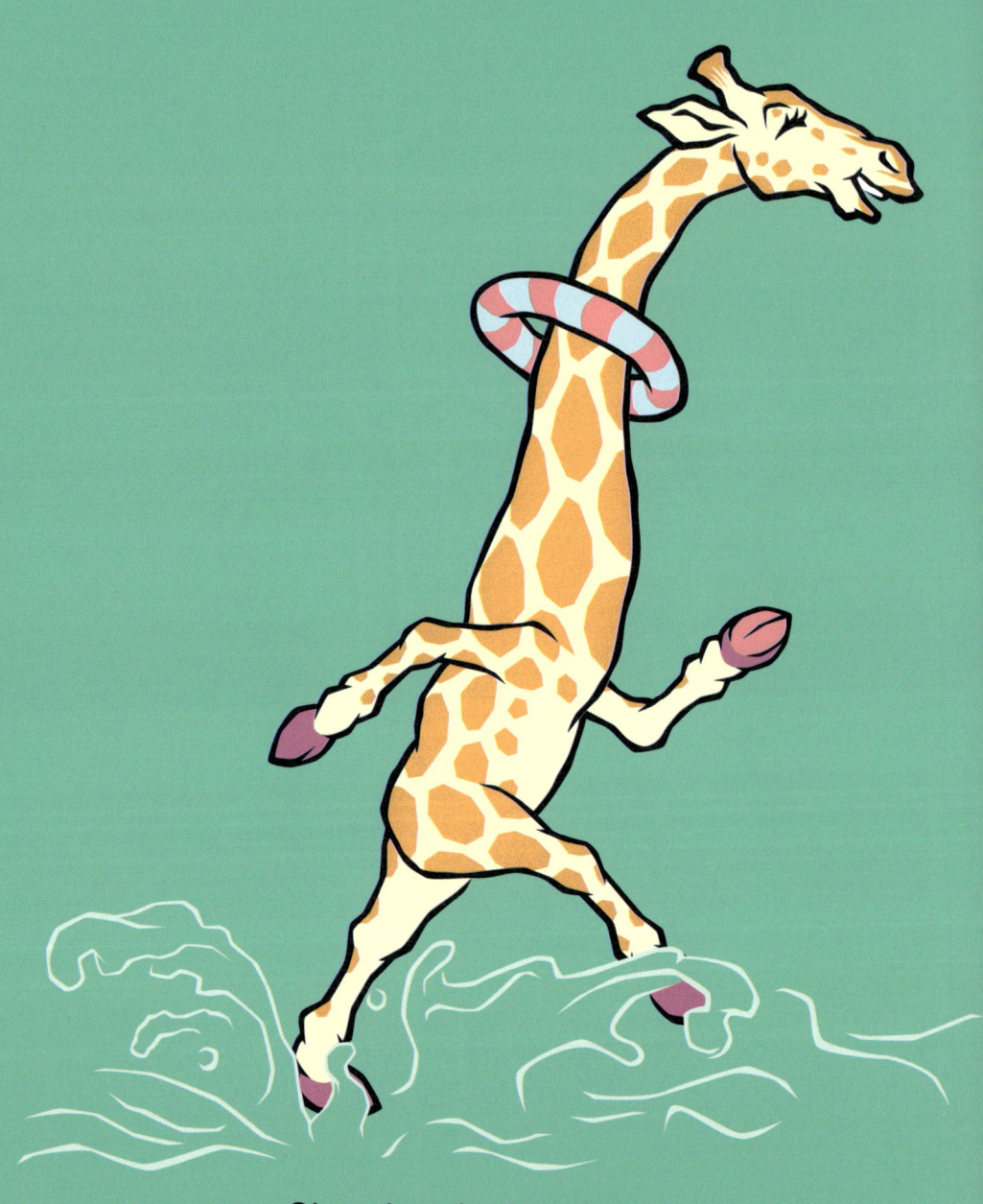

Charging the breakers,
Gerry splashes with joy.

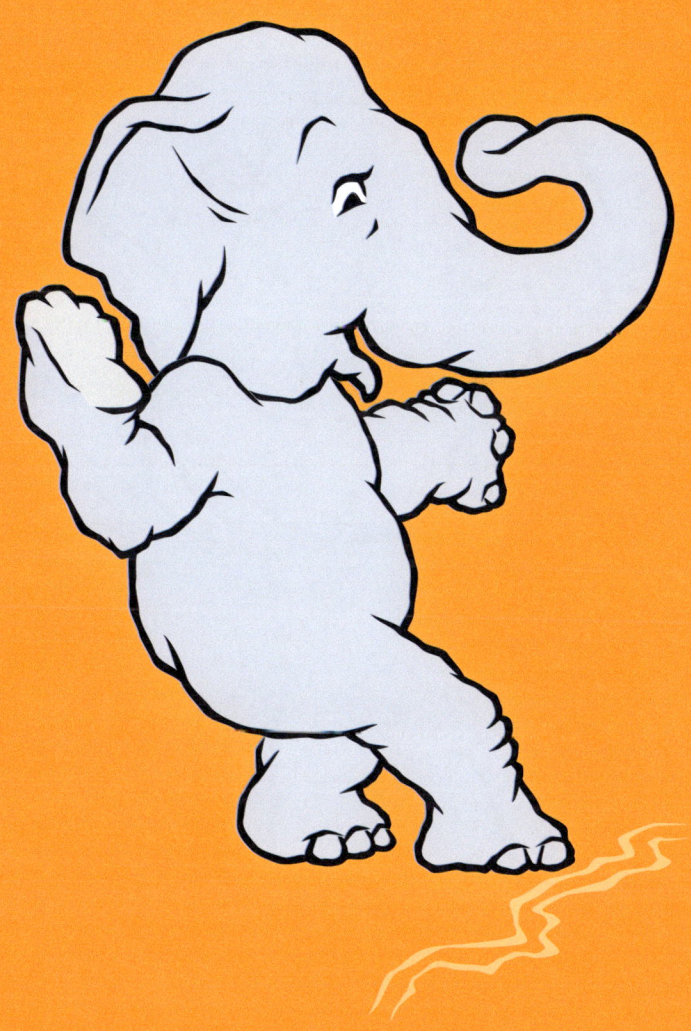

Ellie wades in,
her steps careful and coy.

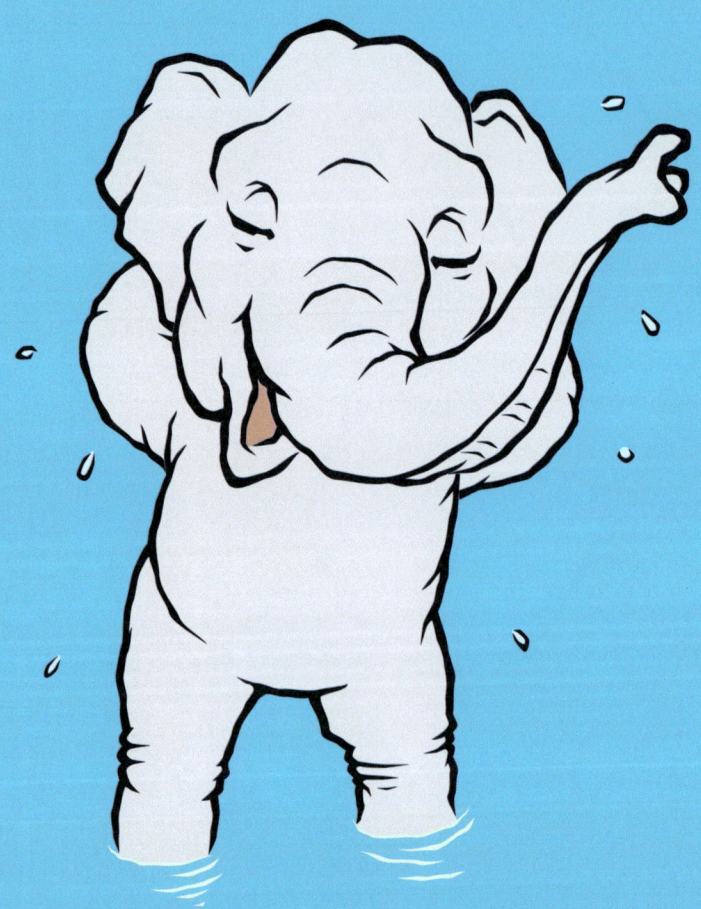

They float and frolic,
each in their way,
until they are ready
to call it a day.

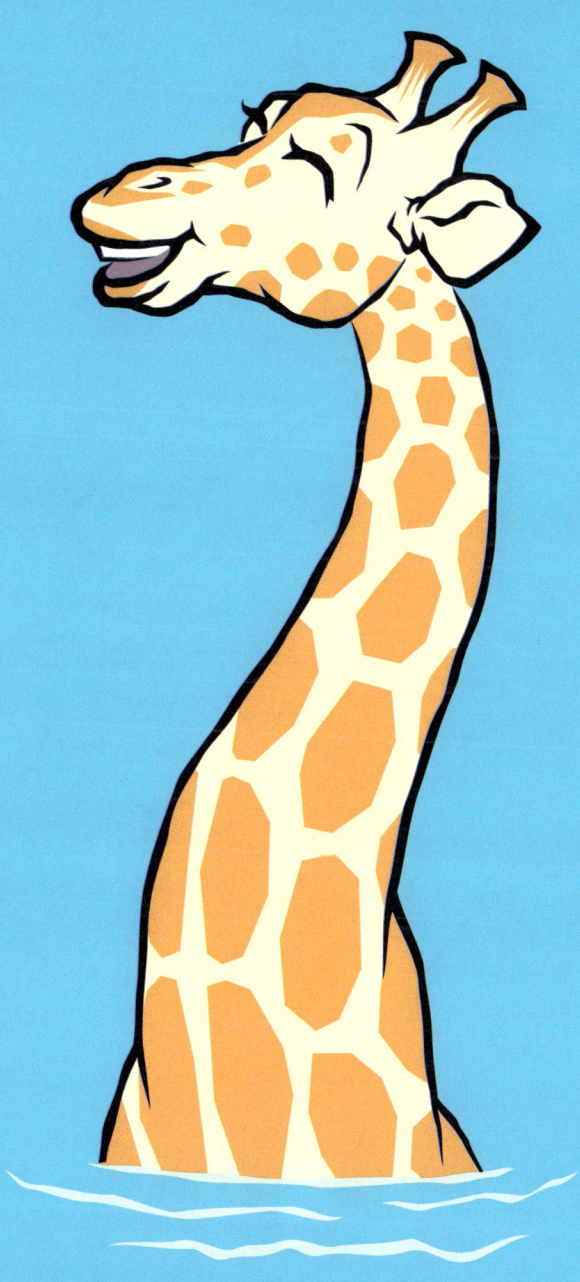

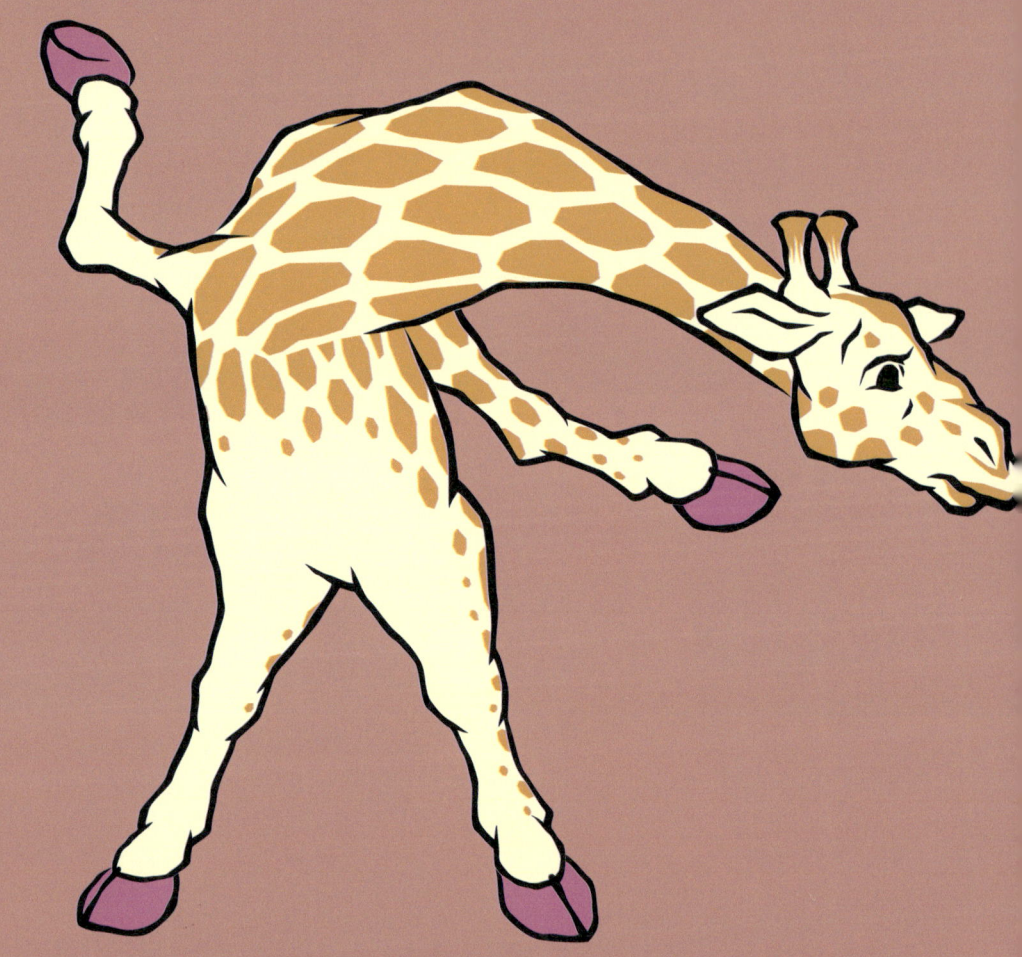

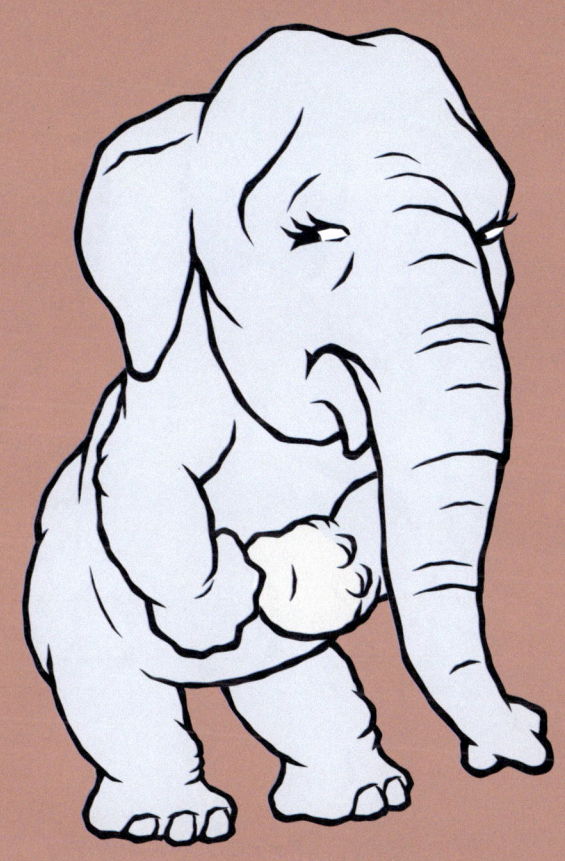

Time to dry, but oh my,
no clothes to be found.
Gerry's happy colors
no more on the ground.

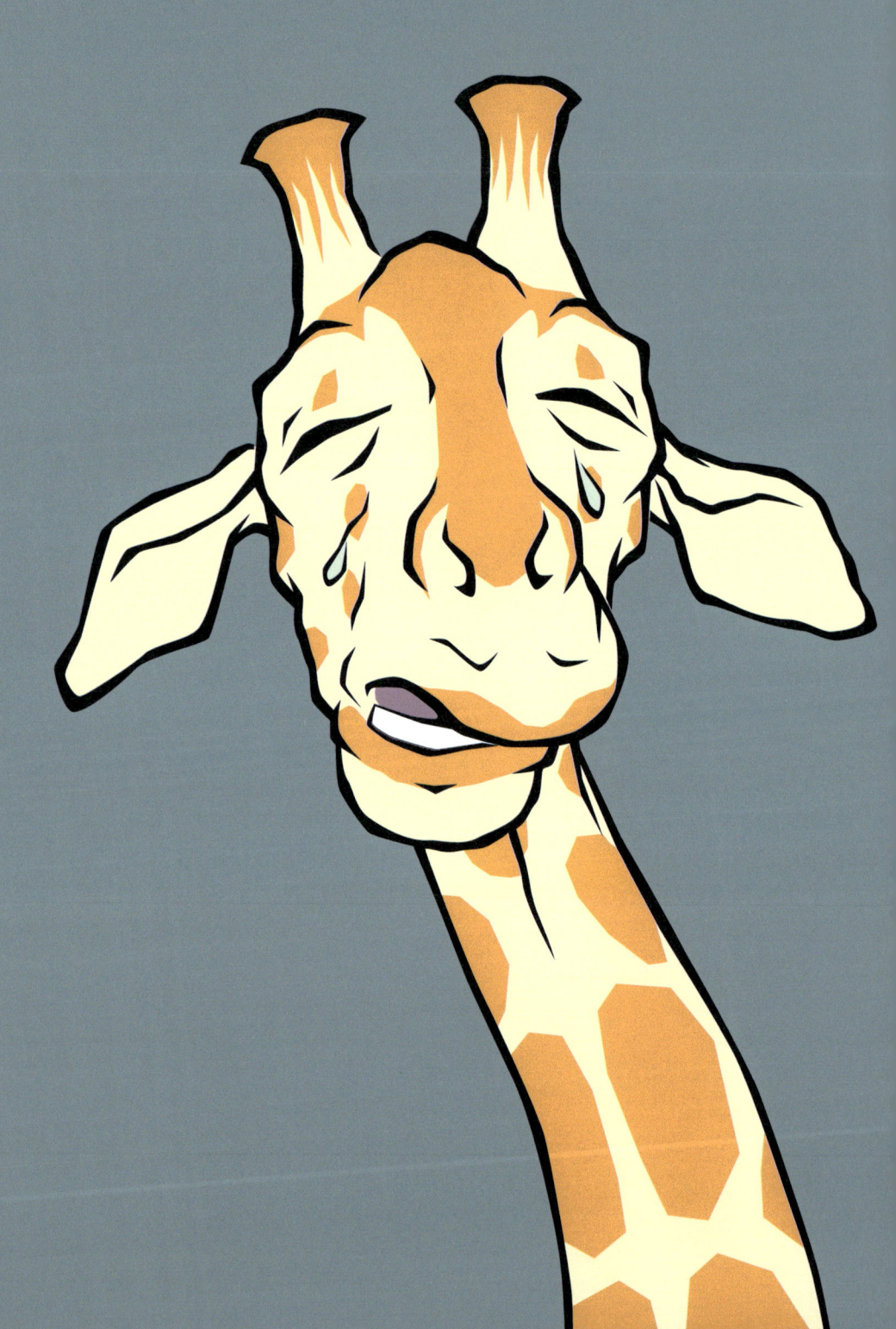

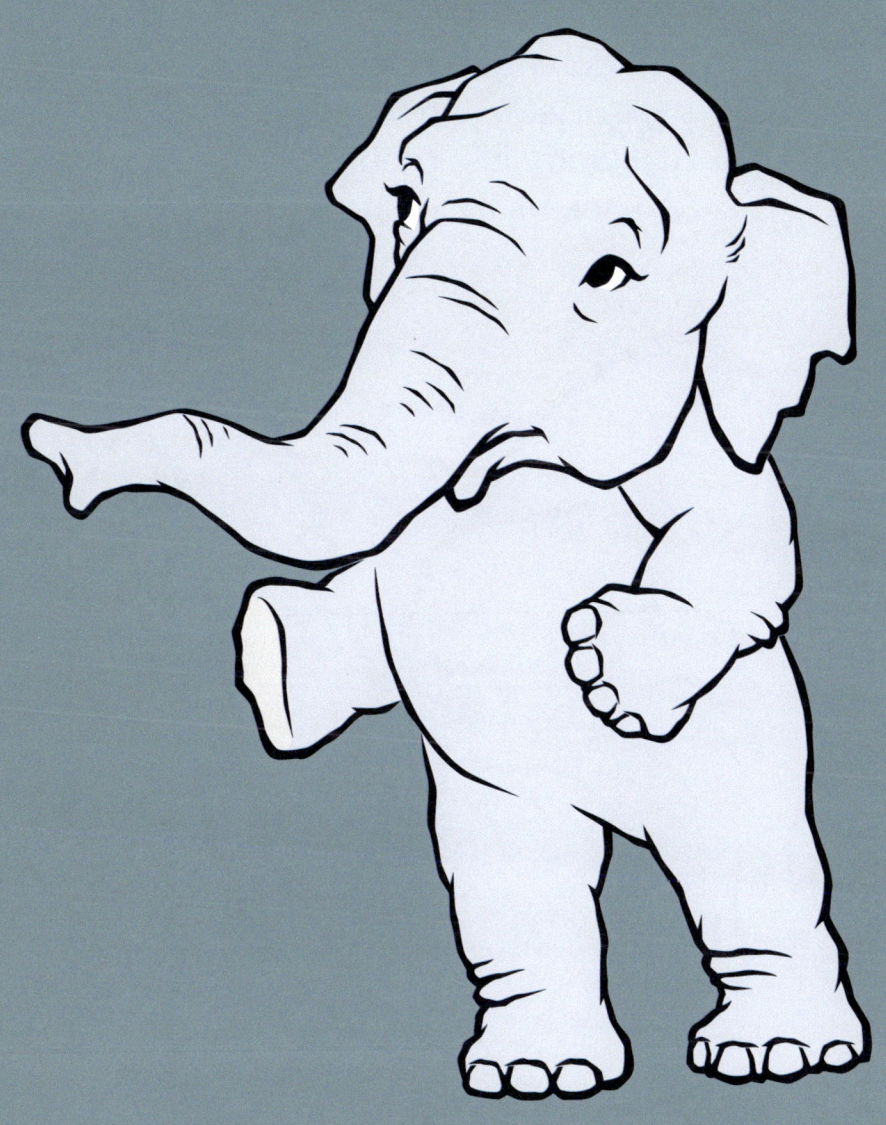

"My clothes are all gone."
Gerry cries in dismay.
Ellie watches her friend
not sure what to say.

"We don't need clothes,"
says Ellie, trying to cheer.
Sad Gerry just droops
and seems to not hear.

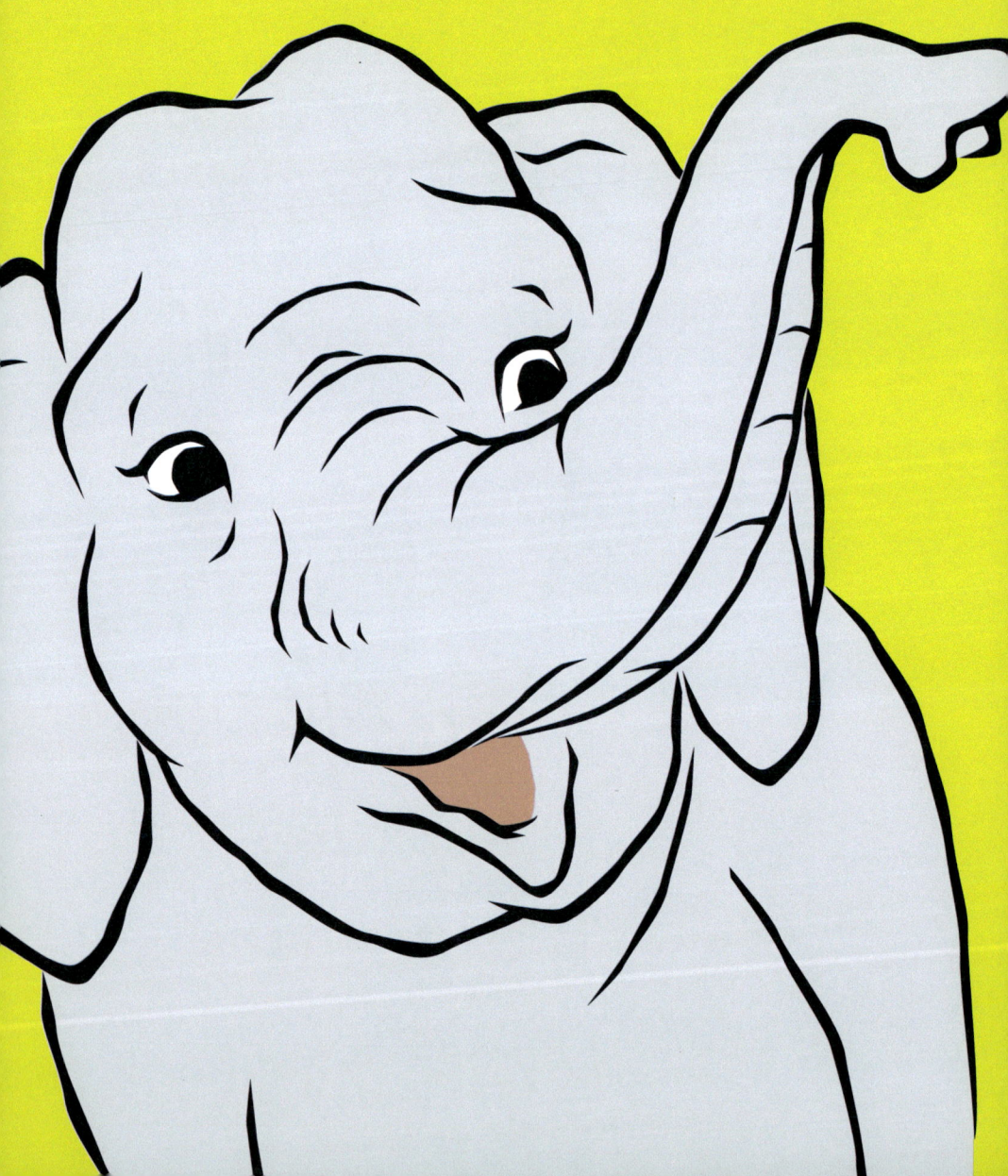

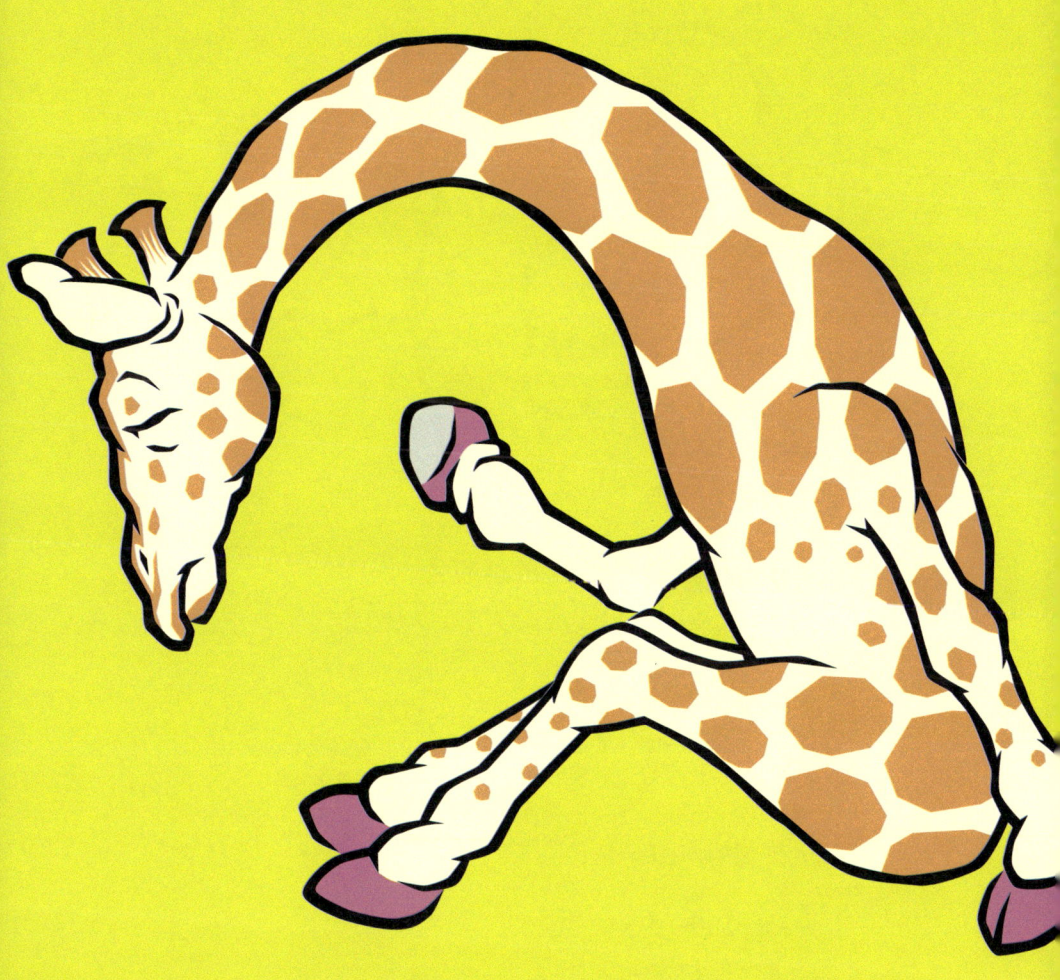

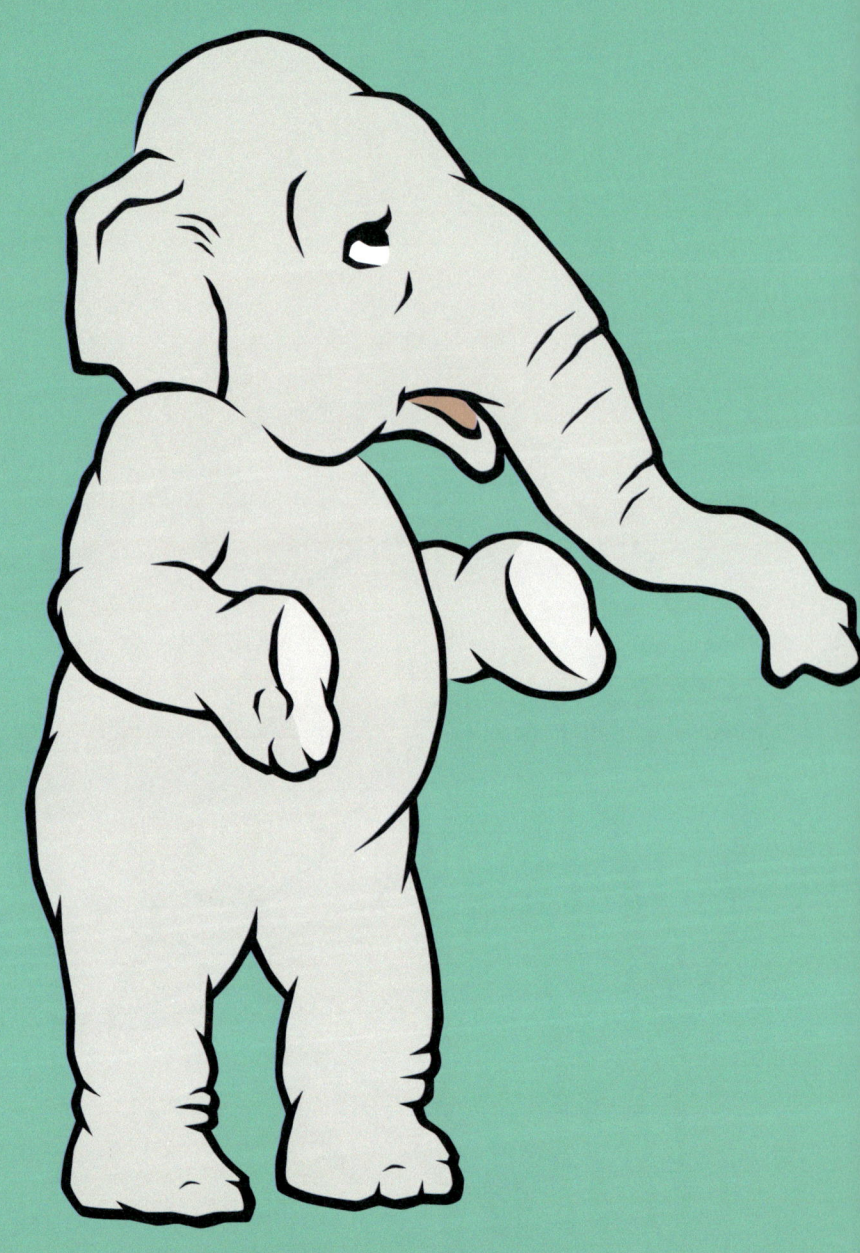

Ellie explains,
"I hate when you're teased.
So I hid your clothes.
I hoped you'd be pleased."

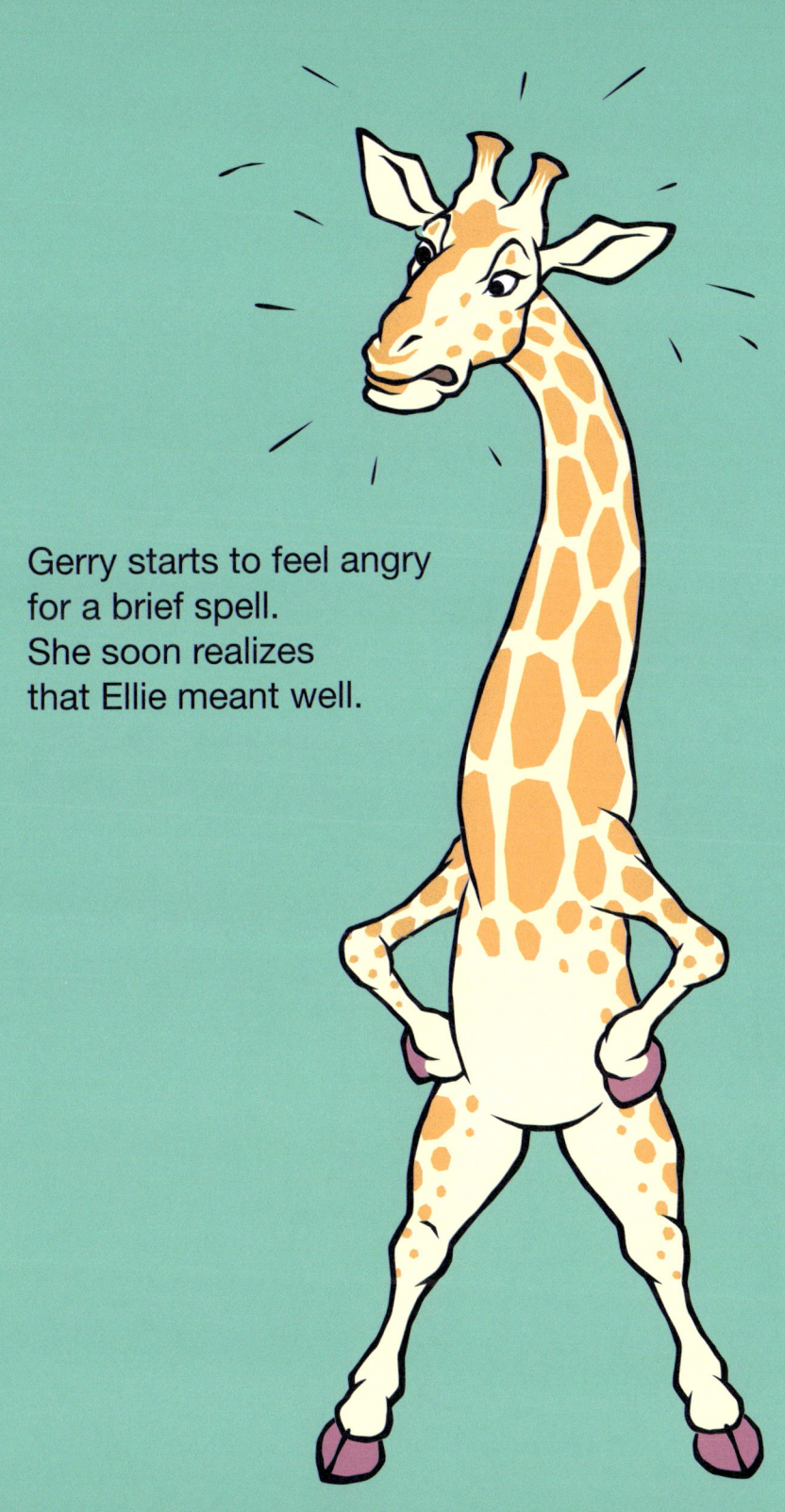

Gerry starts to feel angry
for a brief spell.
She soon realizes
that Ellie meant well.

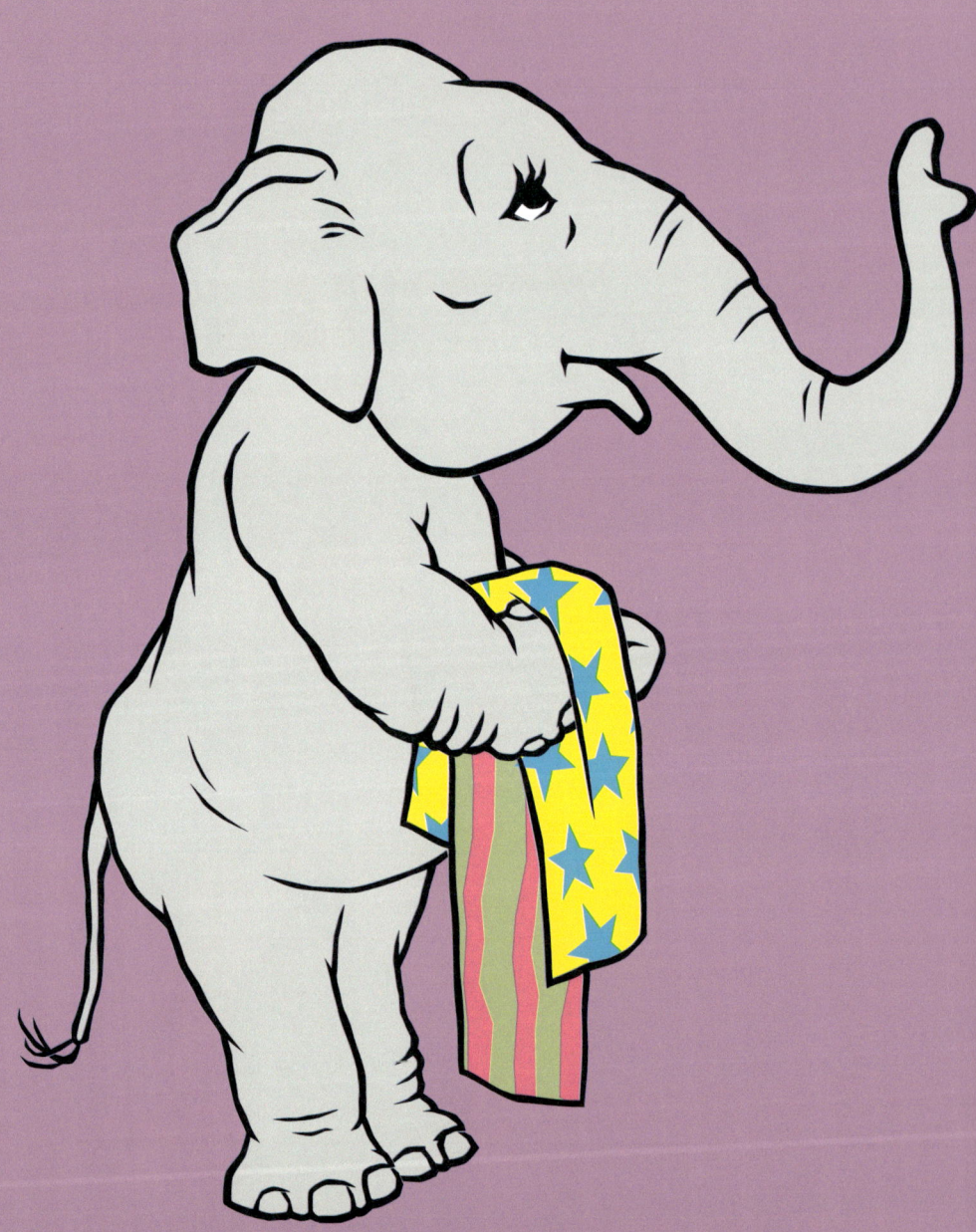

Ellie gives back the clothes.
"I think I understand now."

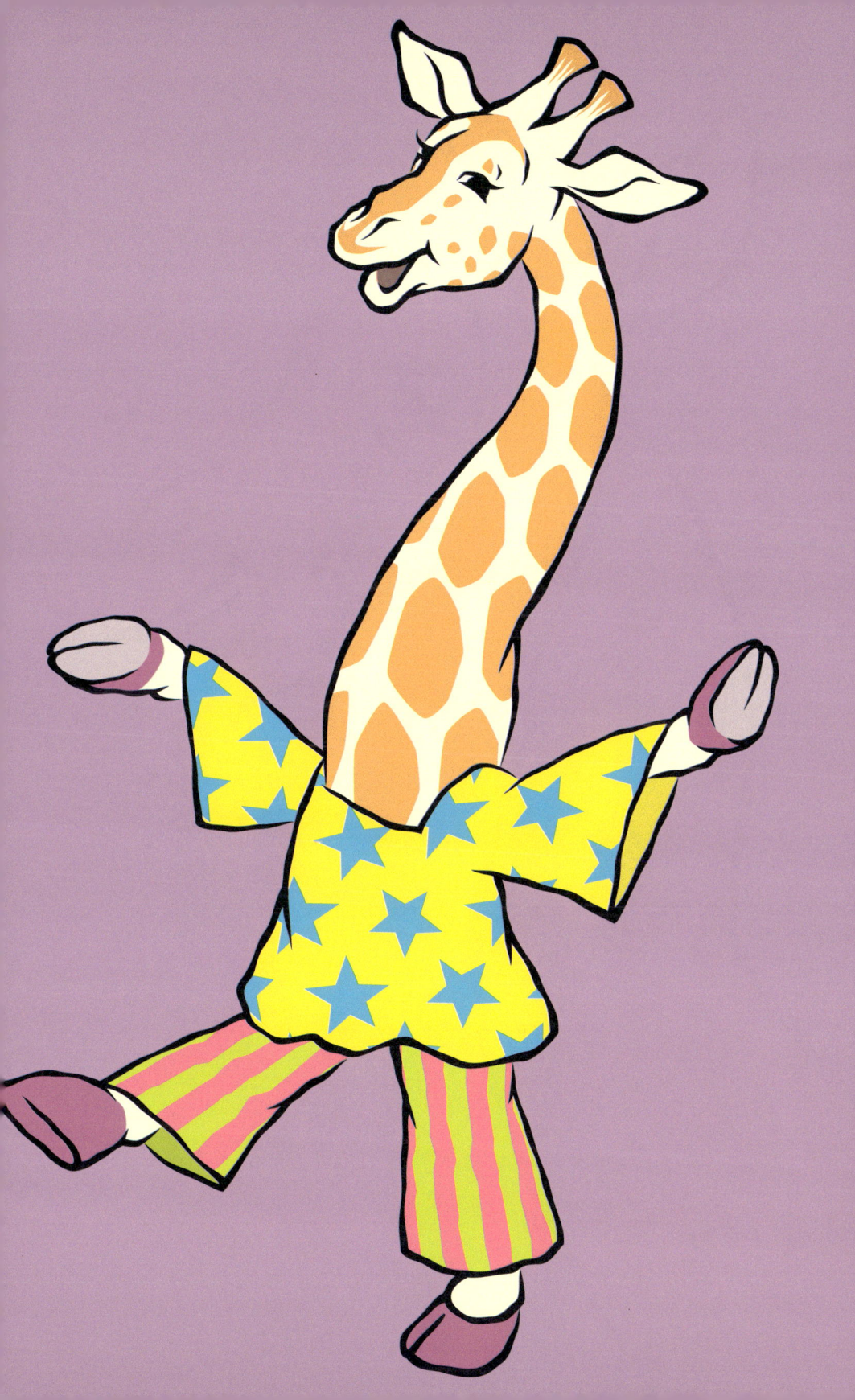

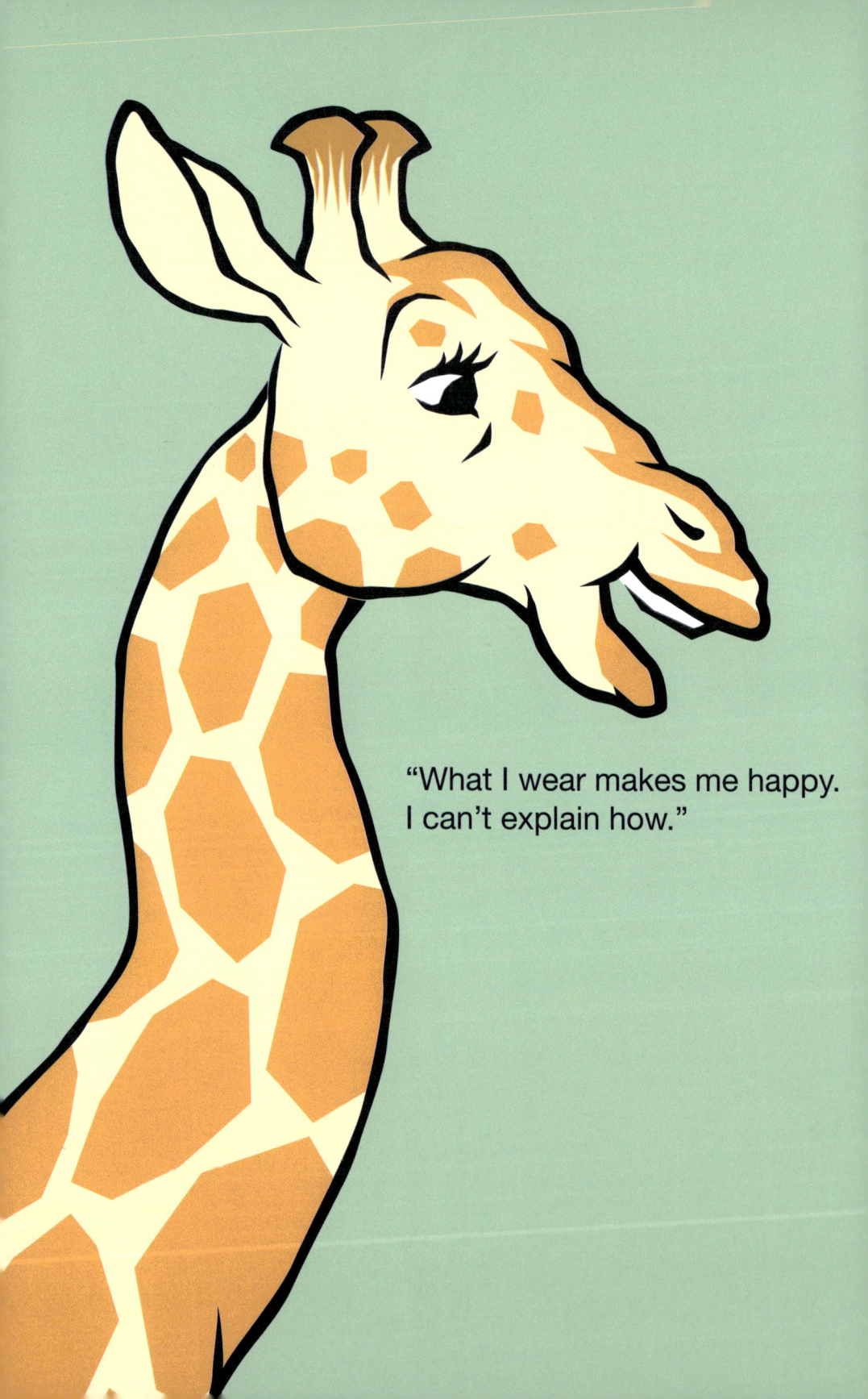

"What I wear makes me happy. I can't explain how."

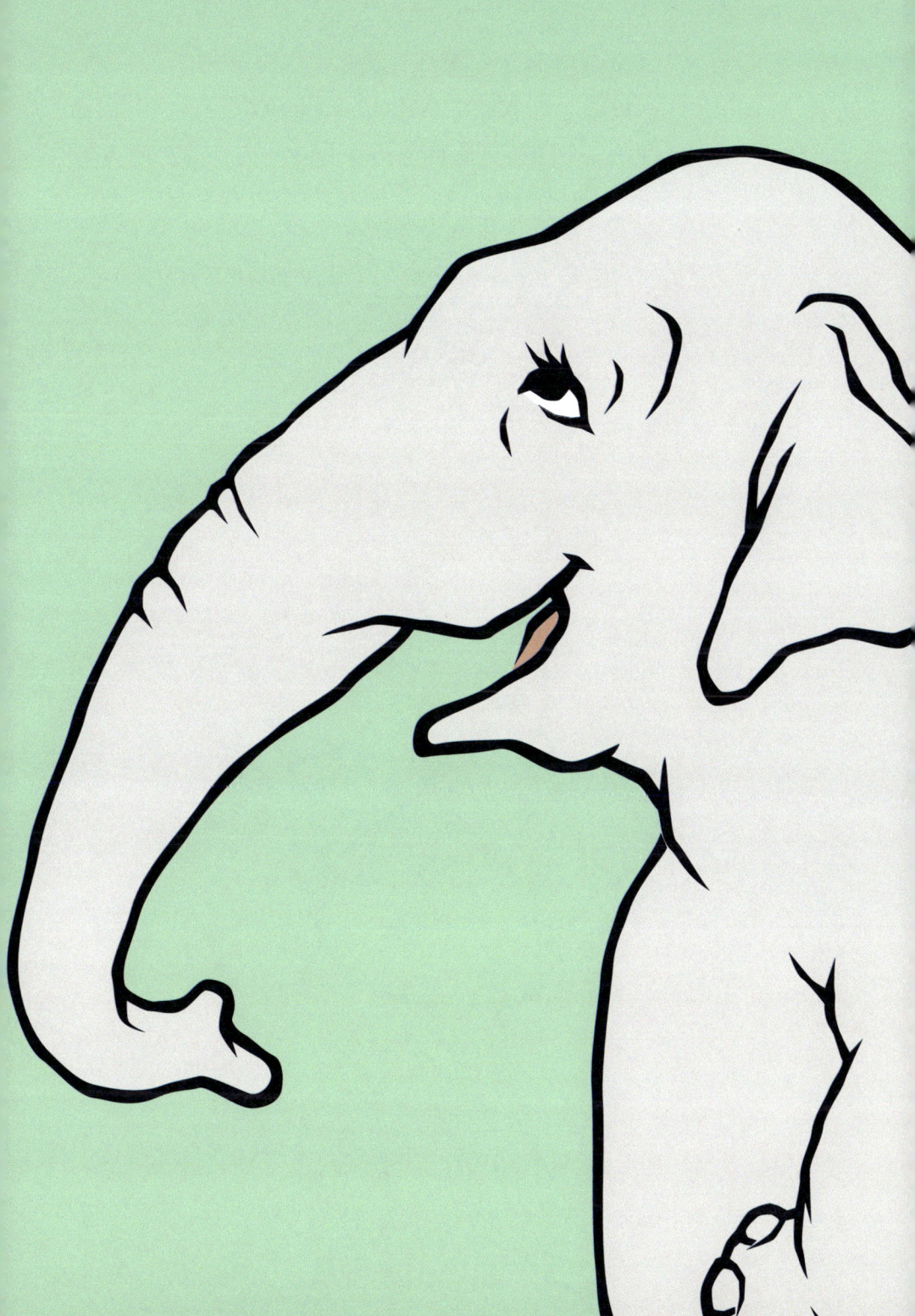

Once Gerry is dressed
she feels great again.
"Thanks for trying to help me
and for being my friend."

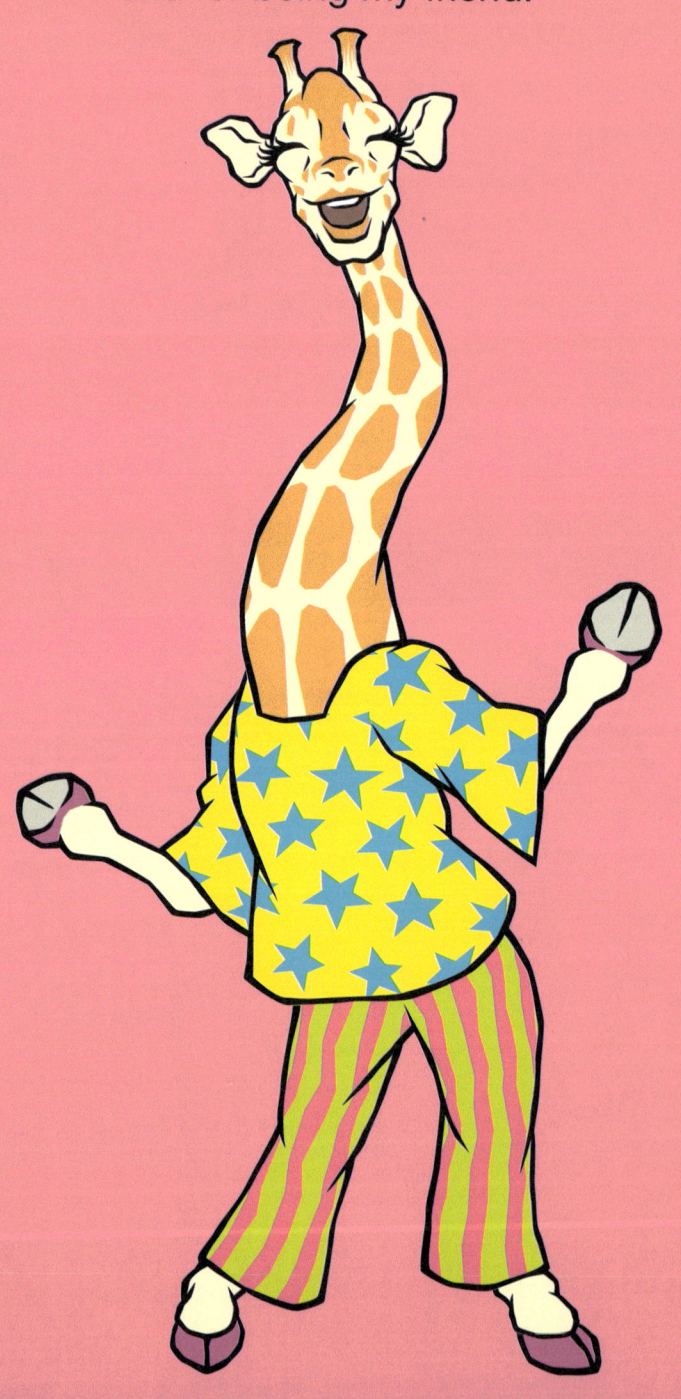

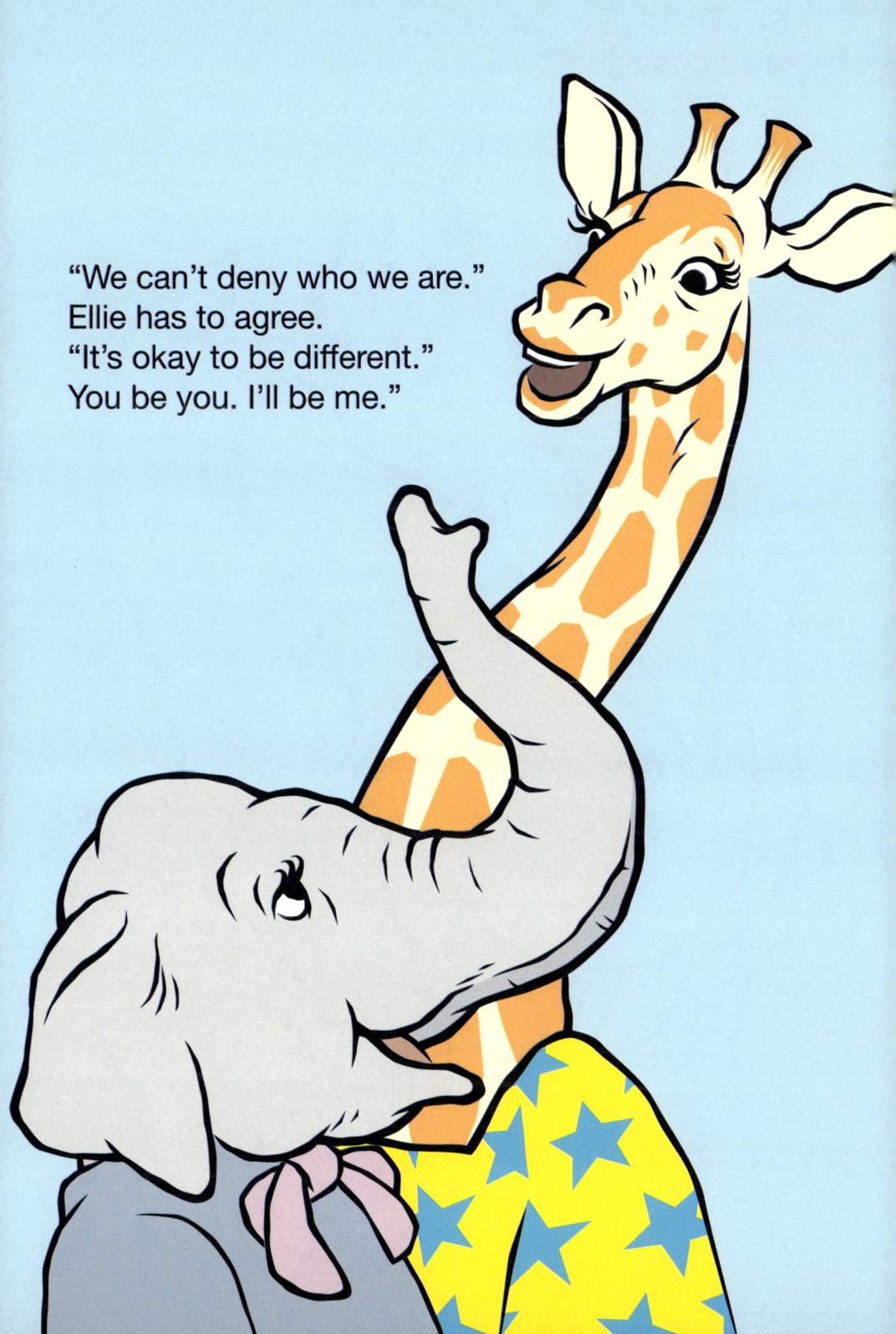

"We can't deny who we are."
Ellie has to agree.
"It's okay to be different."
You be you. I'll be me."

Despite all their differences
great or small,
they find joy in knowing
they'll be friends through it all.

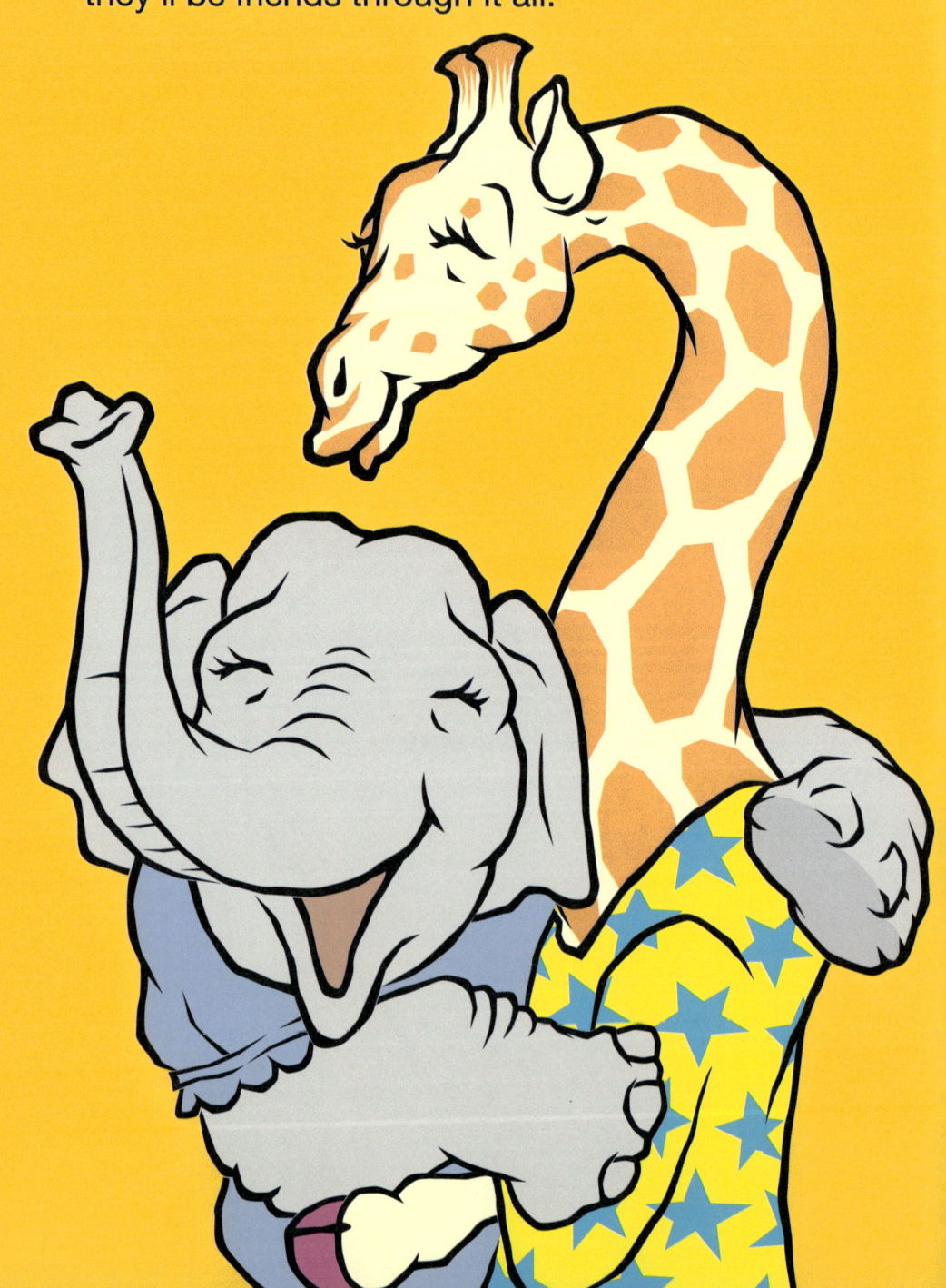

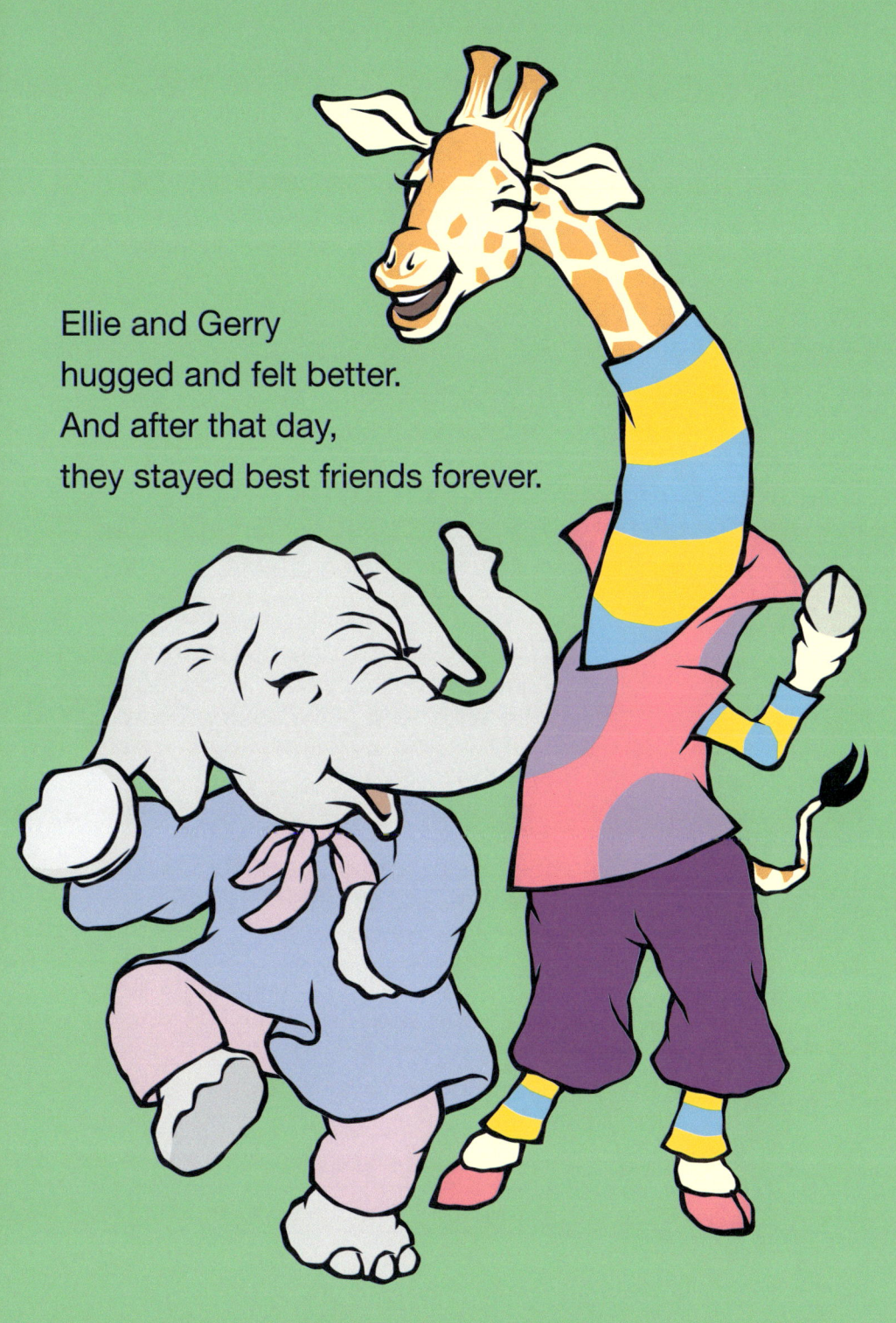

Ellie and Gerry
hugged and felt better.
And after that day,
they stayed best friends forever.

You can't tell a book by its cover. You can't always tell a book by its author and illustrator. But you can tell a book by its readers—or in the case of *Eleanor and Geraldine*, by its original listeners, Lisa and Jennifer Rosenbaum.

Eleanor and Geraldine was conceived by Lisa and Jennifer's father, Jim, as a bedtime story. Jim is a former medical school professor whose scientific writings and essays have been published widely, including in *The New Yorker* online and in journals like *Science*, *Nature*, *JAMA*, and the *New England Journal of Medicine*.

Eleanor and Geraldine has been brightly and whimsically illustrated by a lifelong friend of the author, Doug Katagiri, who was staff artist for the Oregon Zoo in Portland, Oregon.

Eleanor and Geraldine is about friendship, teasing, personal freedom, and acceptance of the lifestyle of others.

Jim and Doug hope that parents and younger readers will enjoy this story.

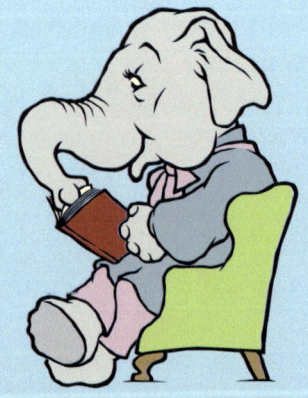

Made in United States
Troutdale, OR
01/18/2025

28109374R00026